TIME
TO
Soar

WHEN LOSS BECOMES
NEW BEGINNINGS

Renee d'Offay

Published in Australia by
Inspire Press
Address: Belmont VIC, Australia
Email: rdoffay@gmail.com
Website: closedcaptions.me

First published in Australia 2017
Copyright © Renee d'Offay 2017

National Library of Australia Cataloguing-in-Publication entry
Creator: d'Offay, Renee, author.
Title: Time to soar : when loss becomes new beginnings /
                    Renee d'Offay; edited by Amanda Spedding.
ISBN: 978-0-9954477-0-7 (paperback)
ISBN-13:   978-1-5448072-3-2 (Createspace)
Subjects: d'Offay, Renee.
                    Deaf--Biography.
                    Hearing impaired--Biography.
                    Deafness.
Other Creators/
Contributors: Spedding, Amanda, editor.

Cover photography by Lindsay Gardner
Cover layout and design by Milos Jevremovic
Printed by Ingram Spark
Typeset by Nelly Murariu at PixBeeDesign

Disclaimer
All care has been taken in the preparation of the information herein, but no responsibility can be accepted by the publisher or author for any damages resulting from the misinterpretation of this work. All contact details given in this book were current at the time of publication, but are subject to change.

The advice given in this book is based on the experience of the individuals. Professionals should be consulted for individual problems. The author and publisher shall not be responsible for any person with regard to any loss or damage caused directly or indirectly by the information in this book.

Praise for *Time to Soar*

"There is a rawness and honesty in the way Renee tells her story. Without fanfare Renee leads you on an insightful, emotional, human journey of tragedy and triumph. Like the chrysalis, Renee emerges from her destructive illness with a determination to soar and embrace her new life. A truly inspiring story told with humour, modesty, and love. There is an empowering, life-affirming message to be learnt from Renee's attitude and approach to adversity."

Rob Walker
Secondary Teacher, Grovedale College

"Renee's story is proof that no matter what life throws at you, it is possible to keep getting up if you have a positive mindset and good people around to support you."

Nat Heard
Assistant Principal, Clairvaux Catholic School

"*Time To Soar* is the captivating and inspirational story of Renee d'Offay. It is a story about loss, courage and love. A must-read for anyone who has experienced any significant obstacle, and could do with a dose of motivation. This book is an amazing reminder that determination and love can overcome life's most challenging hurdles. I dare you to read this book and not be touched by it."

Julie Postance
Author of *Breaking the Sound Barriers: 9 Deaf Success Stories* and Director of iinspire media

"I'm partially Deaf and I think only few people can appreciate the experience of not really, truly belonging to either world – hearing or deaf. I am inspired by the hard work you did to live your life to the max and get the best results. Such a driven person and your book is not only motivating for me and others, it is successful."

Danny Ashley
Electrician, Downer Electrical

"*Time to Soar* is not just a book about deafness, but rather a story about dogged determination and how even the bleakest of events can put you on the path you were truly meant to walk. Renee defines the best part of the human condition – kindness, acceptance, love, and humour."

Amanda J Spedding
Award-winning author and graphic novelist

To Leanne John, who believes, inspires, and loves.

To Jane Kahle, for her selflessness and
dedication to new beginnings.

CONTENTS

Foreword

I grew up in a family that loved British comedy. We were all huge fans of Monty Python and I'm pretty sure I spent my teenage years answering questions with quotes or songs. My all-time favourite had to be the song 'Always look on the bright side of life' from Monty Python's *Life of Brian*. I also know that's entirely not my style of thinking. I wouldn't openly say I'm a pessimist, but my optimism definitely has its limits. I remember thinking, *how wonderful it must be to only see the good things that life's challenges bring!* I also remember thinking people couldn't really 'always look on the bright side', it must be exhausting!

But then I met Renee.

It was following arguably one of the most difficult times a person could go through. I was working as a Teacher of the Deaf at the Grovedale Deaf Facility P-6 campus, and one of my colleagues was telling me about a family friend of hers – a young woman that had contracted meningococcal and had lost her hearing, essentially overnight. Being only new to deaf education at the time, I found myself quite fascinated with what this would mean for her, and the impact something like this would have on a young adult. I'd been working with students who had often been deaf from birth or very early on, but what would the experience be like for someone who had previously had normal hearing? I often asked after this girl and how she was going. Was she well? How was she adjusting to her hearing aids? How was she coping with all of these changes in her life?

In 2005 Renee came to the school and volunteered for one day a week, and I have to admit, I was intrigued to meet this young lady who had taken such a positive attitude to her hearing loss. She was interested in becoming a teacher and looking at working with deaf students. Even early on, Renee always seemed to see the silver linings, and how she could use what she had to help others. She made an excellent role model and worked with students to help them see that they could achieve their goals. She was learning Auslan (Australian Sign Language), and had become actively involved in the deaf community, both in Geelong and in Melbourne. She began playing basketball with the Australian Deaf Basketball Team and threw herself wholeheartedly into her teacher training, fundraising, and building amazing relationships with people around her.

I feel very fortunate that I was one of those people that built an amazing friendship with Renee. Through school and her connections with the deaf facility we became good friends. She also became my most trusted hairdresser, which mostly just gave us an excuse to catch up and talk when we couldn't at work. I studied my Masters of Education (Language Intervention and Hearing Impairment) with Jane – Renee's twin sister – and I watched Renee complete her teacher training with flying colours and move into her Teacher of the Deaf studies. Watching her work with students from different backgrounds and with different needs was inspiring. Her love for her work was palpable and it was open, real, and honest.

When Renee started working at the Grovedale Deaf Facility as a Teacher of the Deaf, I was working at the secondary 7-12 campus, so I sadly didn't get to spend as much time as I would have liked with her in classrooms. But our Deaf Facility teaching team – with Leanne and Jane – was supportive, strong, and we all had our students' interests in the forefront of our minds. Teaching can be turbulent, and ours was that at times, but together we all worked through difficulties and knew we were never alone. I can honestly say that working with our Grovedale Deaf Facility team has been one of the most wonderful times in my teaching career. It doesn't often happen that you get to work with such like-minded and inspiring women who drive you to improve and nurture you as you do. It is something I am eternally grateful for, from the bottom of my heart.

I think that 'wholeheartedly' is an accurate way to describe how Renee appears to approach everything that comes her way. There is never anything that is too hard or too much for her to do for others. However, after knowing her for over ten years, I also know that sometimes her giving nature and her outward optimism and positivity isn't always felt inside. Her struggles with anxiety are not something everyone would see, and many may not notice unless they look below the surface.

This book lays all of that bare. It is honest and open and gives a real insight into the feelings and emotions beneath everything Renee, Jason, and her family and friends have experienced. I have laughed and cried with Renee through many of these times, watching her joy and feeling her heartbreak, but through reading her words and her innermost thoughts I have experienced it again with greater insight than I ever had before.

When Renee first mentioned she was interested in writing a book, I was really excited. This story of Renee's was something I knew would resonate with many people, regardless of whether they had lost something or just faced other challenges in their life. I thought about students I had worked with and what a positive impact Renee has had on them and would have on others like them by writing this book. Showing them how she chose to see her hearing loss as a challenge and a turning point in her life, and to see the potential benefits it could bring as opposed to wallowing in what she had lost.

Renee sees life through a very specific lens. She chooses to see the good and the happiness in situations, and even when it's hard to find that silver lining she manages to make even the greatest obstacles seem like they can be overcome. She inspires me every day and I know that her amazing story will inspire and touch others as well.

Sally Martin, Teacher of the Deaf.

Introduction

Time to Soar was written from my heart and soul with the intention of sharing a powerfully-positive journey while reflecting on a traumatic experience. There are those like myself who have suffered loss from illness that will relate closely to my story, and I'm hoping others may be inspired to see positivity in even the darkest of times.

Accepting change is a matter of perspective, and while I'm inspired to educate teenagers and young adults with my book, there a range of messages within the pages that will resonate with a variety of readers.

Time to Soar chronologically unfolds my life before, during, and after my hearing loss. It is my hope that you, dear reader, will take the positives from change, and look to a brighter future no matter what cards life deals you.

CHAPTER ONE

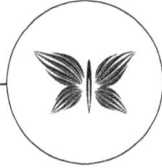

From the beginning

I was born thirteen minutes before my twin sister, Jane, on the 22nd of December 1982. We were a week early and Mum had a reasonably smooth pregnancy, despite growing so big. I was born four-and-a-half pounds, followed by Janey at three pounds, fifteen-and-a-half ounces.

While Mum was pregnant with us, and looking after our fifteen-month-old brother, Brent, Dad was building our first family home in Breamlea, Victoria. So many happy memories were made in this house as well as a few I would like to forget. We do live and learn from these though. These were hectic times for the Kahle family.

During the first months of mine and Janey's lives, there were a few minor complications. Janey went to hospital with bronchitis when she was just thirteen months old, otherwise we settled into our new home as a family of five. Mum and

Dad had planned to have two children, although, as things happen, they were blessed with three.

As kids, Brent and I often joked about Janey being a mistake and an unwanted child, when of course she has been such a huge positive influence in all our lives, especially mine. She's the best sister, daughter, aunty, cousin and friend anyone could ask for. Brent and I would be lost without her presence, her motivation, her kindness, and her selflessness. None of us would change the way things are, especially not me. She has been my rock, my back bone, my best friend and the one to answer all my silly questions. I love you so much Janey.

Mum and Dad had three happy, healthy children and lots of support from family and friends. A special lady, Maureen, who lived down the road from us in Breamlea, selflessly devoted her time helping Mum daily whenever she could; nursing us, doing washing or other household chores, or just being present. Mum and Dad are extremely grateful for her generosity. I don't know anyone else who could share a story like that. What an amazing human being she was, offering her support from the kindness of her heart.

We were (I now fully appreciate) lucky children in a loving family, immediate and extended. We try to share the same love and care with our own families.

We spent our childhood in Breamlea, located between Torquay and Barwon Heads on the Victorian coast, whiling away endless hours and days on the beach, in the sand dunes, at each other's houses, skating the street – wherever we could all hang out for as much of the day as possible. How precious it was being part of a small, close-knit community where you seldom felt alone. We had fresh air, friendships that would last forever, and a place in which we all belonged. Since our childhood, we've witnessed weddings, celebrated exciting milestones together, and been there for each other during the hard times.

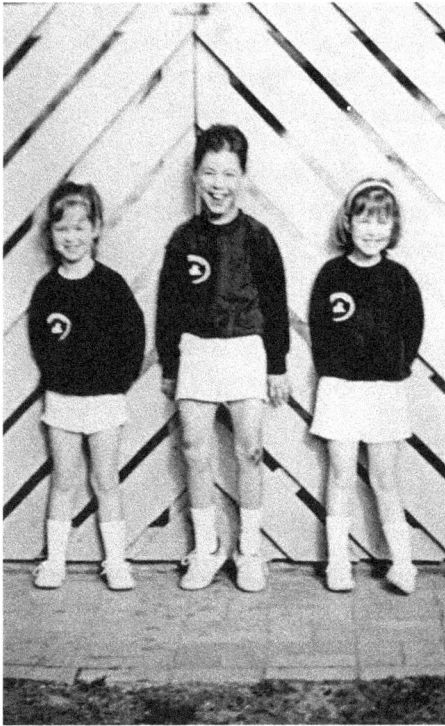

Jane, Brent & I ready for school sports day.

In the early years, we travelled six kilometres each day to the closest school – Connewarre Primary School. At its topmost it had approximately forty-five students. Maybe due to the school's size, there was a tight community feeling with lots of school events, including concerts and family nights. We had different buddies each year and programs that relied on all the students working together. *Last one in the logs*, a game of chase that involved the whole school, consumed many a recess and lunch time, and I'm sure any ex-student could tell you about it. As its name suggests, the last person in the logged area after the bell sent us all outside became 'it'. This saw Grade 6 students supporting preps and the younger kids. I vividly remember one lunch time when my Grade 6 buddy, Daniel Fennessy, piggy-backed me to the area at recess so I wasn't last. These childhood memories still make me smile and feel positive about our experiences as children. While we are all now living in different parts of the world, I'm thankful for access to technology and social media so we can stay in touch, keep an eye on what others are doing, eating, or the places they are visiting.

At the beginning of Grade 5, Mum and Dad decided to move us to Oberon Primary School in Belmont, preparing us to later attend Oberon High School in 1995. A number of families from Breamlea had made a similar decision as it seemed likely that Connewarre was going to merge with other schools in the area due to low student numbers. Our parents were able to carpool to and from school with other families, sharing the travel around their own working commitments. When we began high school, we travelled on the Barwon

Heads bus from Breamlea. This provided opportunity for new friendships, presented us new responsibilities and helped shape us to become the people we are today.

In our late teens, we'd sometimes feel trapped and isolated in Breamlea, despite being surrounded by friends the same age. There was only the caravan park and general store, nowhere else we could meet up at and hang out. As we were growing up, finding our places in life, our friendships extended beyond the sand dunes and wetlands, we wanted to share our community by stretching it within our new groups of friends as we grew into young adults.

School buses were and still are the only form of public transport coming in and out of Breamlea, therefore when we got older we didn't even have the option to escape Breamlea like our friends in surrounding towns did. That feeling of wishing we lived elsewhere pales into insignificance compared to how I feel now – having a connection with a place I will always call home. I love visiting Breamlea; it's calming, peaceful, and a place where I can always fully relax. I now am so thankful I grew up there and hope to be a part of it for a long time, to share it with my children who can then share with their own. Breamlea is now the resting place of three very important family members, and in the future it will be my place of rest along with other family members. This has made Breamlea an extra special location for us to visit often.

As we got older, we pushed boundaries, made mistakes like most children becoming young adults, but our life lessons came from these experiences. We were exposed to great habits and quickly learnt (sometimes from older kids in the community) what was right and what was wrong. Jane, Brent and I were very fortunate to have a range of opportunities in all areas of life, from being in different sports groups to learning how to drive and being responsible. We all played basketball, teeball, swimming, spent years learning to play the piano and a range of other activities. The life Mum and Dad provided is one I hope I can provide for my own children in years to come. My parents are two of my best friends because of their parenting decisions, their commitment to our lives, and their love.

Growing up, I always wanted to be a hairdresser, mainly because of the lovely women who worked where we had our hair cut as kids. I was always so intrigued by the salon, and helped out at the basin when my family were getting their hair done, following the hairdressers around like a shadow. One day I wanted to be just like them.

This was how I saw my future, but we all need stepping stones, right?

My aunty and uncle managed the Breamlea Caravan Park General Store, so Jane and I spent some weekends working in the shop – which we really enjoyed. In Year 10 I began my first serious part-time job, thanks to my friend Leah. She'd recently started working at a fish and chip shop in Torquay, *Flippn' Fresh* and one day at school she told me the owners were looking for more casual staff.

"What do you do?" I asked.

"Just batter and fry the fish and chips," she said.

Sounded easy to me; I had some customer service experience and a happy attitude.

I phoned and spoke to Lyn, one of the owners, that following Saturday after running the idea past Mum and Dad. Lyn told me she was busy as she was on her own and asked if I could go in and see her later that day. A week or two later I started work. It didn't all run smoothly, but despite draining a whole fryer of oil on the floor one night, I still kept my job. Well into my adult life, I remained close friends with Lyn, her husband Don and the family, taking away far more than the skills of cooking fish and chips.

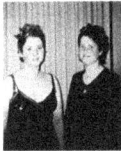

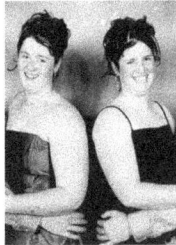

1999, Year 11 Formal. 2000, Year 12 Graduation
Jane left/ Renee right

Before we began high school, Mum and Dad asked for Jane and me to be put into separate classes so we could create our own friendships and find our own identities. This led to us being in different house groups and gave the chance to be as individual as twins could be. During Year 12, we were drawn back together with a common room as the main location where we spent our time with all the other students in our year level. It was after Year 12 that our friendship took on its most positive transition, leading us to inseparable hours and constant contact regardless of where we were.

Janey and I were two of the bigger girls in our groups of friends and year level, but it wasn't until we were in Years 11 and 12 that we recognised our weight was becoming a problem. It was a problem because we were uncomfortable in ourselves, we had low self-esteem, and we struggled slightly in our friendship groups. We were unhappy in our bodies and were at an age (soon to become eighteen) when friends and boys were very significant in our lives.

We both finished our schooling never having had boyfriends. Don't get me wrong, we had boys who were our friends, and we had plenty of crushes (famous ones including Dean Cain and Jonathon Taylor Thomas), just nothing serious with anyone. We got through our final years at secondary school in this particular way.

When I was in Year 11, I completed a pre-apprenticeship in hairdressing one afternoon a week for ten months, at the Gordan TAFE. This contributed to my VCE pathway and gave me a real taster for working in a salon. Despite being offered an apprenticeship at the end of 1999 – after completing Year 11 and the VET course – I went on and completed Year 12. Mum and Dad encouraged me to finish, pass, and receive my VCE certificate explaining to me, "It might be something you need later in life."

(Does anyone else have parents who are more often right than they are wrong?)

Following their advice, I stuck out Year 12 and began an apprenticeship at Radical Waves in Torquay at the beginning of summer in 2001. I really enjoyed diving into the workforce despite missing 'schoolies' with my friends, who all enjoyed their extended time off. Life started to take off. I drove myself to work, earned a regular income, and was learning the basics in the salon.

Though I still hadn't had a serious relationship, I'd started to explore the dating scene and enjoyed going to the Eureka Hotel every Thursday night with my friends. At this time, I was always the designated driver. I had very little interest in drinking due to my new-found love for health and fitness.

It was around this time my physical appearance changed along with the rest of my life. Jane was accepted into Deakin University in Warrnambool where she spent her first year studying for a Bachelor of Arts degree, travelling home most weekends, while I was working in the salon as a first-year hairdressing apprentice. During that first year, I decided to change my food choices and exercise habits, and that started to create some big changes in me. I joined a local gym with my cousin Karen and began my fitness journey – my relationship with my body changed for the better.

Every time I saw Janey, she was surprised at how I looked and asked what I'd been doing. The kilos were literally falling off me, and because she was away during the week (sometimes for two weeks at a time), she really noticed a difference. While she was a few months behind, we were ALWAYS (still are) completely in sync – if one of us did something, it wouldn't be long until the other did. So it didn't take Janey long to change her habits to become healthier and start losing weight too.

People around me, friends and family, started to notice the changes, often making comments that had a positive impact on my self-confidence. Now I look back, I wish my relationship with my body had matched the positive glow those on the outside experienced. Instead, at thirty-four, I'm still practicing appreciating who I am and the body I have so that when I have my own children, I can pass on these positive attributes. I know life isn't perfect and nothing is ever one hundred per cent positive all the time, but it's obvious to me now that only I can change the way I feel, and that starts with me loving me.

At the end of 2001, I had my first proper boyfriend – a twin friend I'd gone to high school with. Because I'd already known him for years, the groundwork was done and our relationship set off on a new path. He was doing a chef's apprenticeship at the Torquay Hotel while I was doing my hairdressing apprenticeship. Our relationship lasted four years during which we went through some challenging times together as well as achieving some milestones in one another's company. As we continued to pursue our lives, each doing the things we loved, he was drawn to New Zealand for a season of work and snow. After we'd tried to keep things going long distance, our relationship ended amicably near the end of 2005.

I'd made my mistakes, learnt a variety of skills, and grown into a young adult ready for the workforce, decision-making, and enjoying life.

CHAPTER TWO

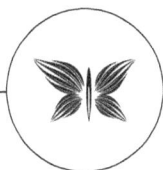

The weekend

Friday

On Friday the 10th of August 2002, Jane and I were feeling happy, socialising at a friend's twenty-first birthday party at a local indoor cricket club. Neither of us was drinking; we were just there to catch up and have a good time. Suddenly something within me changed – I felt dizzy and had a stirring sensation in my tummy. I told Jane I was going outside to get some fresh air. I stood outside for about fifteen minutes near some bushes feeling really light headed, and like I was going to throw up. When I went back inside, Jane asked me if I was OK and I told her I wanted to go home.

> *Janey: On the Friday night Renee and I went to a friend's birthday celebration. We both weren't really drinking, just wanted to show our faces. At one point during the evening Renee went out for some fresh air*

*because she wasn't feeling well. I didn't think much
of it until she returned. When she came back inside
she looked very unwell. Her face was blotchy, as if
she had scarring from severe acne, which wasn't the
case. I was really worried. We headed home and she
went to bed.*

Jane drove us both back home, trying to keep me occupied and awake by talking throughout the whole trip. When we arrived home, I left everything in the car for Jane to bring in, climbed the stairs, got myself a bucket from the laundry and went to my room. I undressed, set my alarm to wake for work the next day and climbed into bed with little idea what was going on in my body. Eventually, I fell asleep.

Saturday

When my alarm woke me early the next morning, I knew I wasn't well. The pains in my tummy were slightly worse. When I moved, every joint in my body ached like I had never felt before. And I had a headache; a very definite, pounding headache. I slowly made my way to the phone in the lounge to call my boss so I could tell her I was unwell and unable to work – receiving the response I was dreading. I had to go to work to cover the appointments I had booked. I thought, *I can't*, at the same time thinking, *but I have to.*

My first client rang and cancelled not long before she was due to arrive and my next appointment just didn't show up. No-one was going to book any more clients in with me as I wasn't in a good way. I walked around the salon looking as if I'd had too many drinks; I couldn't walk straight. I felt completely out of it. Imagine if I'd had scissors in my hands that day! I was an accident waiting to happen.

Maybe my illness was more serious than I'd thought. I waited around out the back, hoping for time to pass quickly. My final client was a friend and was more than happy to cancel. In fact, she wondered why I hadn't called, and was far more concerned about my wellbeing than her regrowth. That day I did no hairdressing.

I set off for home, and after stopping two or three times feeling like I might throw up, I was happy to have made the fifteen-minute drive home safely. I'd driven really slowly with tears rolling down my face. Pulling into the driveway, I didn't care where or how I parked. Within minutes I was in bed.

From this point on, the details of what happened start to blur.

Later on that Saturday afternoon, as I was feeling no better and was continuously complaining about increased pain, Mum phoned the after-hours medical centre in Torquay. The doctor on call suggested meeting us at the clinic so he could check my temperature and a few other things. He diagnosed me with a virus, told Mum to keep an eye on me for any changes – including a rash appearing – and prescribed me some Panadene Forte. After collecting the script and all those wonderful 'Mum' remedies for when you're sick (lemonade, dry biscuits etc.) we went home and I went straight to bed. Mum continued to check on me, looking at my skin, taking my temperature and making sure I wasn't dehydrated.

Betty: During the day on the Friday I had been shopping in Torquay and seen a friend who said that their husband had been very unwell with a flu-type illness for a number of days, and we had also heard of others with similar symptoms. On the Saturday afternoon, I thought Renee should see a doctor so I phoned the Torquay Medical Centre and arranged to visit the doctor on call. When he examined her, he asked all the appropriate questions about vomiting, her temperature etc. Meningococcal meningitis was a concern at the time so he considered this, checking if Renee had unusual spots on her body or was photophobic. He offered her antibiotics and pain relief and told us to keep an eye on other symptoms. For the rest of the day and evening, she took her medication and fluids, otherwise sleeping all the time. Before I went to bed I checked on her again, and there had been no change.

Sunday

It's hard to remember waking on Sunday morning, despite all my attempts to connect the pieces in the puzzle. I was in immense pain – a type of pain I'd never before felt. My head was pounding; I've never experienced a migraine, but I know regular sufferers and feel terrible for them going through such pain – it makes me recall that morning.

I remember Mum coming into my room first then Dad and Jane. They were all talking to me and each other, asking questions and I had no idea what was going on, what they were saying. The look of concern on their faces was frightening. I wondered if I looked different, could they see something I hadn't noticed? Had I physically changed? I couldn't really think or communicate clearly, everything was so blurry and I couldn't hear a thing. It was as if I wasn't in my own body but watching my life from the outside with no volume.

All the natural hearing in my ears had gone. Disappeared. Wiped away. Vanished. Overnight.

From Sunday the 11th of August, 2002 our lives changed forever. *Our* lives, because while it all happened to me, while I personally experienced the loss, it was never going to be the same for my family either.

At the same time as observing this rush of fear from my family, I knew things were bad but I hadn't fully registered my inability to hear what they were saying. My pounding head, aching body and the constant feeling of nausea were controlling the little ability I had to focus on what was happening.

Mum phoned the doctor we had seen on the Saturday and we met him in Torquay again. Armed with a letter from him, Mum drove me to emergency room at the Geelong Hospital. She phoned home to tell Dad, Jane and Brent to meet us there.

When we arrived, I just made it through the first set of sliding double doors before I collapsed into a vacant wheel chair. Not long after, I was moved to a bed in one of the emergency rooms. A doctor and a few nurses floated in and out, offering me water and other things I might need, and

Mum and Dad stayed close by. Dad held a bucket for me but there was nothing in my system that wanted to leave.

The next thing I remember was waking up in ICU.

Betty: The next morning when I went into Renee's room she was sleeping, which I felt was probably a good thing. When Jane got up and asked how Renee was, I decided I should check in again.

She wasn't very responsive. I looked for any tell-tale spots on her body, though I didn't find any. When I asked her questions, she indicated she couldn't hear me and that alarmed me. I began wondering if this was a symptom of the flu-type illness our friend had had, so tried phoning them to ask but there was no answer.

I decided to phone the doctor again who organised to meet us at the surgery in Torquay, once again examining Renee - keeping in mind the possibility that she had meningococcal meningitis. Because he was unable to determine anything conclusive and her hearing was affected, he said he wanted me to take her to Accident & Emergency where the on-call ENT could be called to examine her.

Once we'd arrived, a nurse, Leanne, attended and checked continually on Renee's condition until a doctor was available. After examining Renee, the doctor removed me from the room to talk to me about her condition. He said that he felt she could in fact hear and it was merely an attention-seeking ploy.

I immediately started thinking, don't I know my daughter? Am I so disconnected? Do I not really understand my daughter well enough to miss this behaviour? *These thoughts lasted only a couple of seconds and I asked for a second opinion. The nurse agreed with me when I said it wasn't in Renee's nature to act that way, and there was something more serious happening. (That doctor was never seen working at Geelong Hospital again.)*

The head of the emergency was called in and after very briefly examining Renee, he sent her straight to ICU and said that anyone who had been in contact with Renee during the last twenty-four hours should go to hospital for preventive medication. This doctor diagnosed her with meningococcal meningitis.

Janey: Have you ever felt hollow? Like half of you is missing? From the moment Mum and I woke Renee on that Sunday morning I felt like I had been hit by a bus or sliced in half. I'll never forget the scream coming from Renee as she tried to communicate with us. She couldn't hear a thing. As Brent carried Renee out to the car I stood there, speechless, helpless, and empty. The next few hours I waited beside the phone. I kept checking our home phone was working, making sure there was a dial tone. I was desperate to hear what was going on.

It wasn't until later that night, when Renee had been admitted to ICU with still no definitive diagnosis, that immediate family and those who had direct contact with Renee were called in to the hospital to take a precautionary medication. I tried to call Brent several times, but he was at home asleep and didn't answer. Renee's partner at the time had alcohol in his system so couldn't drive, so I picked him up in Torquay then went to wake Brent. They both needed to take the medication.

My hollow feeling did not subside the entire time Renee was in both the ICU and a general ward in hospital. Eventually, when the feeling did decrease it was replaced by others. It's impossible to explain, but everything about my relationship with Renee (what she meant to me, how I viewed her, the person she was etc.) was different, and still is to this very day. And probably always will be. She is precious and she is my world!

Brent: *I remember it like it was yesterday. I got home from a mate's house and asked Mum what was happening. She said Renee wasn't feeling well and was asleep in bed, but she didn't want to wake her. Later, Renee woke and couldn't hear anything. We had no idea what was happening.*

Next thing we knew Renee was in hospital. The first doctor told Mum that Renee was attention seeking! All of us knew that wasn't in her character, it was something she'd never do. Luckily, a nurse hinted to Mum that she was entitled to a second opinion.

Renee was moved to intensive care and we were
called in to take some medication to prevent it from
happening to us.

I still remember wanting to confront this doctor
face-to-face and have a crack at him for saying
Renee was attention seeking. What a load of shit!
The next day I was working by myself and can
remember crying, wondering why it had happened
to her and what was going to happen next. Why
her? Could it be fixed?

By the end of Sunday, I'd been moved to a bed in ICU
where I spent a few days and then into a general room for
the remainder of a week.

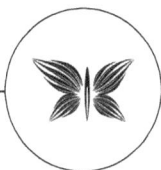

CHAPTER THREE

Hospital

N one of us enjoys going to hospital, but at some stage in our lives we, or someone close to us, will need special care.

My memories are vague about the time I was in Geelong Hospital in 2002. My only real understanding of that time comes from others, and even then I have to take their word for it. My time in ICU only felt like twenty-four hours, not days. I'd wake up, everything would be dark, and then I'd fall asleep again.

The most frightening moment was when I woke inside an MRI machine. I'm positive I would have been awake going in, but I don't remember anything about that. I do, however, remember very clearly waking up inside, not knowing where I was and overwhelmed with terror. I banged frantically on the walls to be heard and was hysterical when I came out, where I was comforted by a nurse and removed from the room.

After my stay in ICU, I was moved into a private hospital bed where I spent a week. A week that felt like a lifetime. I was rarely alone in this room, even at night. Doctors, nurses, specialists, family, friends and many other people filled my room with information, love, support, cards, flowers and most importantly – presence.

Some things stood out for me. One day, a group of medical students came into my room with a doctor. I was lying on my bed with ten adults standing around me having conversations, taking notes, making eye contact with me and each other. It was bizarre. I didn't communicate with anyone; I felt like an animal in the zoo being observed in her enclosure.

As they were leaving, one of the female students wrote on the corner of the white board that had been bought to my room so I could communicate with visitors: *I like your nail polish* and added a smiley face. We made eye contact, smiled, and she walked out. I still wonder what on earth that group of students achieved by visiting me.

The minutes and hours went by but I still wasn't completely aware of the impact from the illnesses and the damage that had been caused. I couldn't hear – that much was obvious. But I hadn't realised how permanent this was.

But as I said before, I was surrounded by positive support. So many people visited me in hospital. I could have opened a florist with all the flowers, and there were so many cards with such beautiful messages. My family and I received phone calls, text messages and 'get well soon' cards from people we had met just once or hadn't seen in years. I was touched and humbled by the number of people who reached out to us, and it helped us to stay strong, soldier on, and accept our new way of life.

While drinking in all this positive energy, I was undergoing testing again and again. Hearing tests, scans, MRIs. I remember putting the earphones on for the third time, slowly becoming more aware of the world around me, wondering if the results were ever going to change.

On Wednesday, August 15th, we were informed that the natural hearing in both my ears was severely damaged and was highly unlikely to return. I had to learn how to communicate differently.

While some people experience temporary hearing loss, I wasn't going to be so fortunate. It was hard for Mum explaining this to me. What parent wants to tell their child such a thing? And it made me feel guilty, it ate away at me. I felt bad that Mum felt bad. How much it hurt her to tell me I'd never hear naturally again was apparent in the tears glistening in the corners of her eyes, and the trembling of her lips as she tried to form the words. I wanted that moment to end so I didn't have to observe mum's heartache.

Janey: I remember the day like it was yesterday. After a few days in ICU and watching Renee lie helpless in a hospital bed, it was the last thing we wanted to hear. She'd been through test after test, scan after scan, and despite the professionals explaining what had happened, true understanding will always be a mystery.

How can you go to bed unwell and wake up with no natural hearing, stone deaf?

They took Renee on the Wednesday for what they said was going to be her final hearing test. While we sat and waited for her, we could only hope for some answers about why it had happened and what was going to happen next. No one could have prepared me for the shock of the news. It is still so vivid. "She will never have natural hearing again."

I was devastated. At the time, we put on brave faces. She was still ill, still confused and yet amazingly positive. I don't know anyone stronger than Renee. Up until this point, I had only read such horror stories in the news; it's not something you think will happen to the closest person to you. The sadness and helplessness I felt floored me. I couldn't escape and I had to be brave. I had to be strong, at least while in the room.

Leaving the hospital that day I knew exactly who I wanted to see. I wanted to hug Amie, Karen, Leah and Don – to cry on their shoulders. Friends and family were the rock that kept us smiling.

In a world of silence, there wasn't much more to say. Of course things moved forward, options were presented and we began a new path on the journey unknown. But we did this together; I wasn't alone. Mum, Dad, Jane, Brent, doctors, nurses and specialists... in different ways, they guided me and kept me informed and supported. There were so many things we didn't know. So much for us all to learn.

CHAPTER FOUR

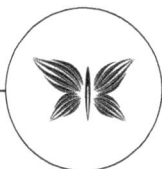

The road to recovery

When I returned home from the hospital, some of my life was the same - the stairs to my house, my bed and my family. Yet so much of my life was completely different. Challenging days, weeks, months, even years were ahead of me. However, due to sound advice and plenty of practice, I now hold a relationship with change that makes it not necessarily a bad or negative thing. Change can be good, right? Most of the time 'difference' is just that, and nothing more. Especially when it's completely beyond our control.

We're all different, and I say that as a twin to a beautiful person who is so much like me but dissimilar as well. It's how we, as individuals, deal with change and difference that makes us who we are. When some people discover I'm deaf they often say straight away - with a tone in their voice and a look on their face - one of two things; "No you're not." (Like I'm joking about it.) Or, "Wow, that must be so different!" Yes it is, but it's that difference I am learning to live with that makes me, me.

I've never wanted people to feel sorry for me or to treat me differently. I've gotten used to most of the change, and so have the people in my life. It was hard for my family and friends watching me go through such a change, and experiencing change in their own way as a result of what happened.

But I don't want anyone to feel sorry about my loss. If I can embrace it and get through the tough times, I want everyone else to as well. *Tough times don't last – tough people do!*

Late last year while visiting my gran, she looked at me with a sadness in her eyes and said how sorry she was for me that I had to live the rest of my life with such a huge change. Of course, it isn't something you would want even for your worst enemy to experience. However, I've recovered. I've dealt with it. And I'll be happy if I live a long and healthy life, filled with laughter and more change. I was given a second chance to take on the world, and here I am, sharing it with as many people as I can, doing something I never even dreamed of doing. Certain people are dealt difficult cards; I was one of them and I have worked hard to not let anything get in my way.

Day One back at home is strong in my memory. I'm not sure why – perhaps it's because it was my first experience in my normal surroundings after losing my hearing. I recall everything from when I woke that morning. I went to the bathroom, which was right next to my bedroom. After this brief stop, I continued down the hallway using the walls to help me balance and keep me upright. Due to the damage caused to my inner ear where there are connections with balance nerves, my balance was affected. It took quite some time to recover and has never returned to normal. I discuss this in more detail in another chapter. As I turned the corner to the main entrance of the house, I ran into my Auntie Lorraine who was vacuuming the floors downstairs. So much flew into my mind:

> *I can't hear the vacuum cleaner. How long has this been going on?*
>
> *I am recovering from being very sick and need rest, but it doesn't matter what anyone else in the house does. A heavy metal band with thousands of fans could fill our house and I'd still get enough rest.*
>
> *I could ask her to turn off the vacuum so we could talk, but it wouldn't make a difference. I still wouldn't be able to hear her.*

In case you're wondering, I'm far from the perfect sleeper. Silence doesn't necessarily give you a pass to peaceful sleep every night. Despite being profoundly deaf, there are very rare occasions where I'm actually in silence, and silence isn't the magic answer for a perfect night's sleep.

Over time, I began to adjust to the way things were, and my other senses started working to cover my hearing loss. I began to use my sight and the ability to feel some of the things people with natural hearing can hear. It was all just so new. After understanding how the change had impacted me,

I began relying on my vision far more than I did prior to this change. From generally noticing more with my eyes to being more inquisitive to what I could see around me. As well as my vision, the feel of things in my surroundings such as doors closing or people walking nearby was heightened from the loss/change. I have discovered that floor boards are a good surface as the vibrations of footsteps are stronger than say those on concrete.

So now, that heavy metal band would probably keep me awake with vibrations and movement – but I don't intend testing that one out!

Mum and Dad had bought a big white board on wheels from Officeworks and put it in my bedroom while I was in hospital so people could 'talk' to me while I was in bed. Whenever I wasn't in my room, I always had a notepad and pen with me. From small talk to big, ongoing back and forth conversations, this was my newly-discovered way of communicating with my friends and family. Rather than always writing, I often voiced my responses, much louder than normal, unaware of the volume. I had to learn the difference between a whisper and a shout by the feel of my voice in my throat.

During the initial weeks at home, many of my visitors continued to speak to me or hold conversations with others in my presence. When people were talking to me, it was really difficult at first. I couldn't hear what they were saying and I couldn't read lips. I watched and observed as conversations took place around me. The skill of lip-reading was one I developed very quickly and it soon became second nature.

After we had all adjusted to how things were for me, my family and those I saw regularly used less paper and more talking/lip-reading. Understanding conversations became much easier – if in doubt, we resorted to a notepad.

Lip-reading is a unique skill and can be more challenging than you might think. Believe it or not, you can actually go to short courses to learn how to lip-read. Unfortunately, being deaf doesn't automatically qualify you with lip-reading skills. I have a range of friends, including those who were born deaf and others who lost their hearing, and the individual's ability to lip-read varies immensely. However, over time, living in a hearing world and practicing it daily means that when I'm not wearing my cochlear implant or when the environmental noise level increases, I rely on lip-reading. It's a mastered skill, not something I'm dependent upon – I need air and water more – but it's certainly a great support to my daily life.

I got pretty bored at home while I was recovering. I had gotten so used to going to work, hanging out with friends and living my life before I was sick that I was ready to get back on track, so I returned to the salon on a part-time basis with my notepad. I eased back into hairdressing by working fewer and shorter days with limited clients. But I was able to find a sense of normality in my life, which was reassuring after such an impactful change.

I often reflect on this time now, recognising how well I adapted to all the changes and my determination to get back on track to the exact way things were before. I have learnt so much from behaviours and choices I made at the time, with no regrets – I don't see the point in that. I do, however, acknowledge that after all these years and my experiences, I would likely approach the change much differently if it were to happen again.

CHAPTER FIVE

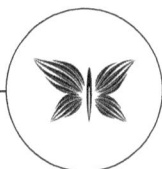

My new life

Life with a cochlear implant is *different*.

It's challenging. It's rewarding. It's not like it was before. But it's something I've gotten used to. It's LIFE!

After three months recovering at home, and slowly returning to work, and after serious discussions and lots of thought, I decided to go ahead with a cochlear implant. This was an anxious, unknown experience for my family and me, but it also seemed reasonably straightforward.

OK, like many operations it involved an element of risk. What stood out for me the most, considering how much there was to take in, was when I was shown by an audiologist about how the internal piece was inserted between the facial nerve and the taste nerve, and into the shell-shaped cochlear. There was a chance that if during surgery either side was touched, there could be permanent or temporary facial damage or loss of taste. It's rare, but it has happened in some cases and therefore is a risk.

I was also quite concerned about getting a new hair style, as when things were being explained to us, the audiologist described and showed where they would shave my head for surgery. I was close to getting a 'number 1' all over! Me having my head shaved – not by choice – felt like a big deal.

The date was set for me to have cochlear implant surgery on my left ear. I chose my left because I'd have better access to sound from passengers in the car when I was driving. There was no other real reason to choose one side over the other.

Roy: It must have been hard for Renee as she was between two worlds – the hearing and the non-hearing. Having had hearing then losing it overnight, how could anyone understand unless they'd been through it themselves? As a parent you want what's right for your children. I never thought Renee would refuse to go ahead with the implant, but in hindsight that was probably selfish. All I wanted was for her to hear again. I didn't consider that she might have second thoughts.

With the decision made, anxiety levels set in. I faced minimal preparation prior to the surgery. The procedure itself involved a day visit in the Royal Eye and Ear Hospital in Melbourne then home to rest for a week, giving the wound the required time to heal.

When I woke in hospital with a bandage around my head, I couldn't wait to get it off and show Janey so she could check how much hair they had shaved around my ear. Of course, in the end it wasn't that bad – only a very small section that didn't take long at all to grow back and was covered by the pieces of hair above. Although I wasn't able to wash my hair for a few days and I needed to rest, the surgery had been successful and my facial and taste nerves were normal.

About a week later Mum and I returned to Melbourne for an appointment with the surgeon in order to check the wound area was healing as expected, and to make an appointment to get the external microphone piece mapped and fitted.

The day I got 'switched on' (as it's known) is another very memorable day in my journey, and one I am likely to always remember. Mum, Dad, Jane and my boyfriend were all there to support me, thankfully.

I'm sure that being switched on isn't the same for everyone, but for me, after having nineteen years of natural hearing, it was a bizarre experience. To begin with I just listened for sounds – tapping a stick on a table when I could hear sound. After having not having heard anything for a few months, and with the difference in sound from the implant, everything felt very weird. I had five sets of eyes sitting around the table watching me, gaining their own experiences of the event.

I then tapped for sounds I could hear that were as loud as I could manage. This helped to design the programs on my processor with each of the twenty-two electrodes or channels I had access to. When the audiologist felt we had created effective programs, I was no longer connected to the computer and could independently rely on my new processor.

Wow! I'd spent the previous three months in silence and being able to access sound again was strange, even stranger as it was so different than before. When others spoke and when I heard myself, it was all so unusual. I didn't expect it to sound the same, but I'd had no idea what it would be like.

At first, I couldn't distinguish much difference between male and female voices due to the frequencies. Voices sounded very mechanical, like listening to Daffy Duck speak. Such an incredible feeling and experience, and one that is difficult to explain. After feeling as comfortable as possible with my new access to sounds, I collected my case of parts, batteries and cords, and we left the hospital. As we walked towards the car park, my next strange experience was the sound of traffic passing by. When we were younger, family friends had one of those cane rainmakers that looks a bit like a didgeridoo. As you turned it up one way, something fell inside that created a sound like rain. Well, to me, that was what the traffic flowing past sounded like, but strangely it still looked the same.

> *Roy: I was so happy for Renee the day her cochlear was turned on. The look on her face when she heard her first sound in months was fantastic – or was it me seeing something I so wanted for her? She was probably terrified but would never let you know. After being close to not being here, Renee sees every day as a blessing. We were beside her, supporting her the best way we knew how.*

Of course, having nineteen years of natural hearing has only ever worked in my favour, never against me. I was able to make use of my prior listening knowledge and experience of hearing, focus on remembering sounds and adjusting to a completely new and unnatural form of hearing. It took some time to get used to the sounds with regular visits to the hospital, which slowly became few and far between.

Years later, I now wait to be called in for appointments. These appointments involve being hooked up to a computer that maps out the twenty-two electrodes I have access to with my cochlear – similar to my initial visit. At first I was adjusting to the softest and loudest sounds by tapping a stick and designing programs to suit. As the need for changes to my program decreased, visits became less frequent. The programs are stored and I go about my daily life with these programs forming my access to speech and sound.

I still wear the original processor (an Esprit 3G, Petunia I affectionately call *Tunie*) I was given fourteen years ago despite there being a number of changes in technology and newer models becoming available. I do have another model, a Nucleus 5 known by most as *Tiny*, however I'm selective regarding when I wear each of them.

Maybe it's just habit and a sense of security that makes me prefer to wear Tunie. She has spent some time in Sydney, on two separate occasions getting repaired (she went swimming in a toilet one time and was saved), otherwise she's well looked after and serves me very well. I shock a lot of people with the fact I still wear Tunie and how well she works.

I accept there will come a time when Tiny will take over, but for now I'm content with them sharing the role of supporting my ability to hear. I needed to name them early on so people didn't ask, "Do you have your ear or hearing on?", but could refer to my specific device. I have no idea if other people name their devices.

Where the future heads as far as hearing technology is concerned, is unknown. I wouldn't change the tough decision I made all those years ago and I'm thankful for what I have been able to achieve with the access I have. I often reflect on what could have happened – obviously the most tragic would have been if I'd lost my life and wasn't around today to write this book. I could also have lost a limb or my sight. I could also have walked away unchanged.

It's a disease that impacts individuals differently, and it hit me hard. It stole my hearing, but it also gave me a second chance at a life I've learnt to love. Although it was a traumatic experience, I have been exposed to many new things, made lots of new friends and experienced a life I would never have had the opportunity to experience had things been different.

Back to work

After a few months at home, I nervously made the slow return to the salon and eventually became a qualified hairdresser. However, everything was noticeably different. Communicating with clients and the other staff with all the environmental sounds of the salon was difficult because I perceived the working environment differently. This made me feel really unsettled.

I'd taken the get-back-to-normal attitude and approach and stuck with it, but on the inside I wasn't happy. So I decided to take a break from hairdressing, look at some other avenues and perhaps try something different. The 'hands in many baskets' approach certainly relates to this time in my life. I tried and tested every aspect of the hospitality industry you can think of. I floated between fish and chip shops, Brumbys and bistro jobs, often doing more than one at a time.

Finally, I decided to do a part-time, local Auslan course with some family and friends. This is where I met a case manager, Nicole. And I was so envious of her ability to sign so fluently. She told me about the Diploma of Auslan at a TAFE in Richmond that she'd studied for two years full time, and I decided to look into it. I applied for a mid-year intake, had an interview, and was accepted to begin in June 2004.

I travelled by train from Geelong, staying with a friend some nights, and loved what I was doing. I really started to learn more about myself and the new person I was, making some fantastic connections with some beautiful people. I embraced life.

An important aspect of this course was attending a signing-only weekend camp hosted by the teachers with deaf and hearing-impaired guests present. This was a huge eye-opener for me as well as a stepping stone to creating some amazing friendships. In particular I met four deaf boys with whom I had lots in common. Thomas, Matthew, Brent and Wes were all very patient with my beginner signing yet so easy to talk with. I learnt that Matthew had a caravan in Breamlea, Wes was an avid Geelong Cats fan, and both Wes and Thomas were keen basketballers. Brent's love for sport and fun saw us click quickly too.

I left this camp a slightly different person, able to switch off more often and really absorb myself in my new deaf world. I kept in touch with all the boys after the camp and intended to see them again, which I did, often. Thomas encouraged Anita, my friend from TAFE, and me to join them at the upcoming National Deaf Basketball Club Championships (NDBCC). I was in awe for another whole weekend, meeting new people who were all competing for the championship title and beginning to feel a part of the Deaf community. This was so cool.

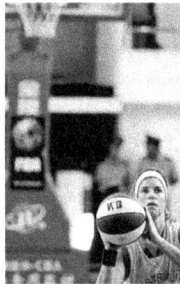

Representing Australia at the
3rd World Deaf Basketball
Championships, 2007

Thomas introduced me to a few of the female players from the Victorian team and it wasn't long before I started playing socially with them at the Melbourne Sports and Aquatic Centre (MSAC). I competed in my first NDBCC in Ballarat in 2006, winning the title for a Victorian side. Not long after, I was encouraged to participate and try out for the Australian team, who were being selected for the third World Deaf Basketball Championships in Guangzhou, China, the following year. I was selected! But I knew I had a lot of hard work and dedication ahead of me. Individual training, fundraising and travelling interstate for training camps started to consume the majority of my life. I was motivated and fully committed to the team with no representative basketball experience but bucket loads of determination.

My family, friends and extended networks were on board with fundraising efforts and endless support. My experience in China allowed me to learn some valuable lessons, and it pushed me to keep striving.

I maintained my commitment competing in the annual NDBCC and was proudly selected for a second chance to represent my country at the 2009 Deaflympic games. This was big! With some positive player and coaching team changes, this Deaflympic journey was one of the most memorable, challenging, and exciting things I've been involved in since losing my hearing. And I had the privilege of leading the team as vice-captain.

Mum, Dad, Janey and Jasey, along with family members of the other players, attended the games wearing gold and green, cheering us on. Having familiar faces on the sidelines got us through some very tough competition, and I really can't express how proud I was to have represented Australia in a game I love. Had I not experienced what I did in 2002, I would never have had those opportunities, and some of the friends I have today.

While I was studying Auslan, I was introduced by a friend to a teacher of the deaf, Leanne, who was working at a local school in the deaf facility. Due to my enthusiasm and our growing friendship, I began volunteering at her school on my one day a week off from TAFE. As my two-year course was coming to an end, I considered my options beyond the Auslan diploma. Most of my friends in the course were going on to become Auslan interpreters, while others changed path completely. I decided to continue my studies and applied for a Bachelor of Education degree – primary. I was accepted at Deakin Geelong (my fifth preference) where I started my degree at the beginning of 2007. At the same time, I also completed a Bachelor in Education in LOTE (Languages Other Than English) Auslan at LaTrobe University, which involved part time study in 2007 and 2008.

At the beginning of 2011, I successfully started my first full-time teaching job at Victorian College of the Deaf (VCD) in Melbourne. I had my very first, small class of students whom I taught through Auslan. This was a very exciting yet challenging year as I adjusted to working full time, travelling by train to and from Melbourne each day as well as studying my Masters in Deaf Education, Teacher of the Deaf (TOD).

While I loved the experiences and opportunities at VCD, the travel had an impact on all aspects of my life, so near the end of 2011, I decided to apply for a position closer to home. I was extremely lucky when a TOD position became available at the school I had volunteered at. I jumped at this, applied, interviewed, and started working there at the beginning of 2012.

Suffering a life-threatening illness sure did change my life, dramatically.

CHAPTER SIX

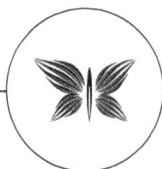

Meeting my soul mate

On a Friday night in October 2005, I was visiting my friends Nicole and Ben at their house in Leopold, a suburb on the outskirts of Geelong. I was doing Nic's hair ready for her 'hen' weekend.

Nic and Jane were both studying for a Diploma of Education at Deakin University, and not long after they'd met, it became the typical two-for-the-price-of-one friendship with us. I referred to her as "Nic, Jane's Uni friend", as I could never say her last name: d'Offay (doff-ay). Little did I know, it would one day become my own.

This was the night I first laid eyes on Jason, Nic's younger brother. When I left, I thought, *Nic has a hot brother.* I'd recently ended a long-term relationship and Jasey was in one so it wasn't something I intended to follow up.

The next day I mentioned to Nic that I thought her brother was very good looking. She responded, "Don't go there", and the conversation was left at that. I thought her response quite strange. On another day she explained to me that Jasey was in a long-term, on-and-off again relationship and it was best I didn't get involved. I didn't intend to pursue it – he wasn't available.

A few weeks later, Nic and Ben's big day arrived. Having met some of the family and friends on the 'hen' weekend, Janey and I were able to relax and enjoy ourselves. I spent the morning in Leopold doing hair and makeup for the beautiful bridesmaids and stunning bride. The morning was filled with laughter, champagne, and lots of hot pink.

After witnessing the ceremony in Geelong's biggest church – St Mary's – Jane and I went home for a shower and changed into our wedding celebration attire. Upon arriving at the reception venue, I entered the area where the bridal party were relaxing before their introduction and touched up the girls' hair and makeup. There was a real buzz. Jasey was sitting and chatting with Brie, one of Nic's good friends and bridesmaids. He said something to her then Brie said to me, "Hey Neighsy, Jas wants to know why you're not putting any makeup on him."

"He's already pretty enough," I replied.

I hadn't stopped to think how that might be taken, and was a bit embarrassed, but no one said anything and we went on to have a great night. I don't recall speaking with Jasey again that night as he was busy mingling with his family and friends and spending time with his girlfriend.

Two of the d'Offay cousins approached Janey and me with an awkward but funny pick-up line that left us all chatting and socialising for the remainder of the night. Jasey later told me the boys had commented to him that it was a waste of time dropping good pickup lines on the deaf chick because she missed them all. This is something we all laugh about now.

Twelve months later, Janey, Angus (Jane's boyfriend at the time) and I were getting ready to leave Geelong for the drive over to Somerville to spend the weekend with Nic for her birthday. As we were packing the car Janey casually said to me, "Did I tell you Jasey and his girlfriend broke up?"

Jokingly, I replied, "Oh, really? Should I put more makeup on?"

We laughed, got in the car and started the two-hour drive around the bay. I'd only met Jasey on a few occasions around the time of the wedding, and one other time at their parents' house in Frankston, but for some stupid reason I felt a bit nervous about seeing him this time.

We met Nic's immediate family at the local tavern for dinner. Jas and I ordered the same meal and when I realised that, I felt like a teenager all over again. After dinner, we went back to Nic and Ben's house, where we were staying for the weekend. We sang Happy Birthday and ate cake. Jasey started talking about snowboarding while I patiently listened. Nic stopped him after not too long explaining that I knew how to snowboard and didn't need all the finer details.

Not long after this, Jasey left to go and stay with his cousins for the night. They were all meeting up with us at Caulfield races the next day. Saturday was a beautiful day. We had lovely weather and great company. Later in the afternoon, Ben and I were chatting and he insisted that Jasey was keen on me. I brushed this idea off. However, when Jasey returned to our area, reasonably drunk by this stage after having had Jager-bombs for breakfast, I was quite nervous. We exchanged numbers... well, Ben gave each of us the other's number. I made a bet with Ben (for a six pack) that Jasey wouldn't call me. The boys stuck together and went off doing what they do at the races, which meant we didn't really see much more of them.

Jasey texted me on the Sunday, we exchanged email addresses and started getting to know each other. For a week this was how we communicated and I'd asked him not to call me so I could win my bet with Ben. In the end, Jasey said he would buy me a six pack, I'd lose the bet but we'd be able to talk.

The Saturday after the races, Jasey made the three-hour trek from Inverloch, where he was living at the time, to Breamlea to spend some time with me. Janey and I were still living at home; however, Mum and Dad were in the middle of an overseas holiday so it was just us.

When Jasey arrived, I was watching *Scream* in my room, which I paused to answer the door. I invited him in then asked if I could finish watching it. Despite the fact he'd travelled for hours to see me, finishing a movie I had seen many times before seemed more important. I think I was just trying to settle my nerves. This guy was hot, he'd driven hours so we could see each other and I was well out of practice with the dating game.

When the movie finished, I gave Jasey a tour of Breamlea explaining what had happened in various places over the years and we really opened up to each other. We started our friendship being very honest, and this is one thing that I will be forever grateful to Jasey for teaching me. That afternoon he asked me lots of questions about my experience with hearing loss and how the cochlear implant worked. When he questioned me about how long the batteries lasted and if I had ever been in a situation without new batteries, I looked at my handbag replying that it hasn't happened often because I have spares everywhere. He was genuinely intrigued about my life in a way I hadn't experienced before, and I was chuffed by his interest. I was beginning to think this guy was a keeper.

Later that evening, I had been invited to a friend's twenty-first and, of course, been given the OK to take Jasey along. I was nervous because lots of people from my past would be at this party and I wanted Jasey to feel comfortable. Funnily enough, we hadn't been there very long, a few introductions and perhaps one drink, when I got warning beeps in my ear to tell me my batteries were going flat. It was so strange considering that only that afternoon we'd been talking about the few situations I have been in with flat batteries and no backups. Even stranger was that while we had been talking, I remember looking at my handbag saying I always carried spare batteries. I searched my bag, Jane's bag, our cars – there were no new batteries to be found!

I gave Jasey the options: we could stay with me not being able to hear or communicate well with each other, drive home and get new batteries then return, or drive home and stay there. We drove home in silence, each lost in our own thoughts.

Jasey turned the music up really loud, laughing about the fact that I couldn't hear to complain about it. I put new batteries in, switched on, apologised for the awkwardness and we both laughed about the situation. As time passed, we decided to stay home, stashing new packets of batteries in my bag, car and anywhere else I could think of.

After replacing my batteries, the first thing Jasey said to me was, "Perhaps I should learn sign language."

I didn't really know how to respond because his kindness was so honest and obvious.

While we agreed we didn't want to rush into a relationship, it wasn't long until we were in love. Something just felt right instantly. Jasey met Mum and Dad within the first few weeks at a family day at the races and our relationship took its course. Even though we'd agreed that we didn't want to be committed as each other's boyfriend/girlfriend, our friendship grew quickly as we got to know each other, and everything felt right. We were open and honest from the beginning so we naturally wanted to be a part of each other's lives as much as possible. Within a month it was official and we had become the VIP in each other's life.

Jasey was already moving home to Frankston the first year we were together, and it wasn't long into this year that he decided to move to Geelong after his twelve-month contract ended. We moved into Janey's first house, living out the back in a separate unit known as the Love Shack.

We both knew what we wanted, but after some discussions we agreed we would wait until I finished studying before getting engaged. We had been together less than eighteen months when one Sunday afternoon Jasey insisted we go to Breamlea for a beach walk. After arriving home from a big weekend in Melbourne, I wasn't keen to get in the car to drive out to the beach, I was more than happy to walk around our home in Grovedale. But he was persistent, and with Janey's encouragement I gave in. (She knew something I didn't.)

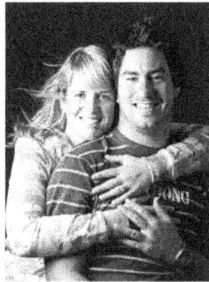

Me and Jas at a photo shoot for
our engagement invites.

We arrived at Breamlea, parked at Mum and Dad's house and Jasey said we would walk first, go in and say "hi" after.

When we reached the lookout at the top of the track, Jasey got down on one knee and asked me to be his wife. I was so surprised but of course I said, "Yes!". We continued our walk around the beach, Jasey sharing the story of purchasing the ring while I had a smile from ear to ear. I was beyond excited I was going to marry my best friend.

Jasey had been ring shopping with Janey and Nic a month or so before and ordered a ring that fitted Janey's finger perfectly. Unfortunately, due to a basketball injury, it wouldn't fit my finger. However, he was still set – I was the girl he wanted to spend the rest of his life with. I'm so glad. Being engaged to Jasey was one of my happiest times. I loved everything about it and eventually (wearing a resized ring) I was able to show it.

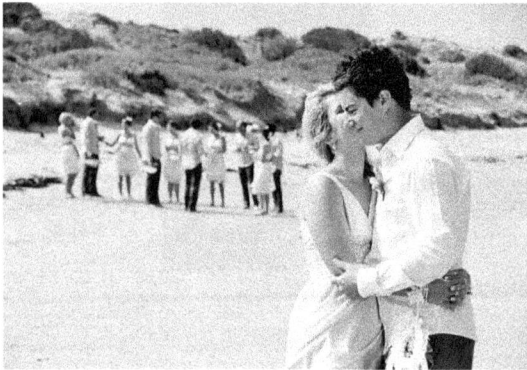

Wedding day - January 9th, 2010.

We wanted a January wedding so we could always go away to celebrate our anniversary, both being teachers and on holiday at that time of year. Almost two years later on the 9th of January 2010, we exchanged vows, said our "I do's" and shared our first kiss as husband and wife. Our wedding day was very special as we celebrated our love for each other surrounded by lots of family and friends.

At first when people asked me, "How's married life?" I felt like it wasn't really that different to being engaged – which I'd loved. As the years have gone by, my response to that question has changed. Being married to my soul mate is by far one of my most favourite things. I'm married to my best friend, a guy who makes me laugh, cry, feel loved, and everything in between.

You have to communicate and be compassionate to make a strong marriage develop. It's not always perfect. Together we have been through so much and as individuals we have been able to support our ever-growing relationship. Jasey has been a huge inspiration to me both physically and mentally. Through his knowledge and guidance I have trained and completed seven half-marathons and one full marathon – distances I never imagined I would reach. Jasey and I have both changed so much during our time together. We understand each other and ourselves with open hearts, open communication, and a shared lifelong goal of happiness. I can't bear to imagine my life without him in it, and I'm grateful for the friendship that brought us together.

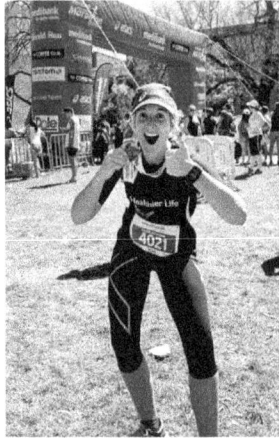

Completing my first marathon in
Melbourne, October, 2014.

CHAPTER SEVEN

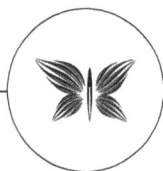

Living with deafness

Living with deafness, and being the only deaf person in your family experiencing the loss of a sense is not as simple as some might think.

Before any of this took place, I didn't know much about meningococcal meningitis. A boy in our area, Zane Henry, had contracted it not too long before me. I knew him through friends, and learnt that as a result of the disease, he'd also suffered from glandular fever. This was temporary but a scare nonetheless for him and his family. There were other cases around the same time, but they were only stories to me, not something I thought would ever happen to someone I know, let alone ME!

My illness had an enormous impact on my life and the lives of my immediate family. I was nurtured and cared for by these four wonderful people more than anyone could imagine.

I still am. They were the air that kept me breathing, the light that kept me shining, and most importantly they kept it real. I became a very different person, and to some extent so did they. Each of their lives changed, too.

I would have considered us a happy, honest, loving and sharing family prior to 2002, thanks to Roy and Betty for bringing us up in such an environment, teaching us good morals and protecting us when we needed it. We were far from perfect; we all had our moments. However, I believe this life-changing experience had a huge impact on the bond within our family. We all needed each other more than ever, we all understood what we were going through (them more than me), and most importantly, we bounced off each other's strengths and support to understand and get through this challenging time.

I would not be who I am today without any of them, and I wouldn't want it any other way. They all make me proud to be the person I am, regardless of how crazy they sometimes think I can be. Yeah, I might have made it through the tough times, but life would not be the way it is for me now without my family. Every decision, every idea, everything I shared with them or wanted advice on, Mum, Dad, Jane and Brent were all there for me, and this will never change. Now Jane and I are over thirty and we still call each other for advice, and we all rely on each other's support.

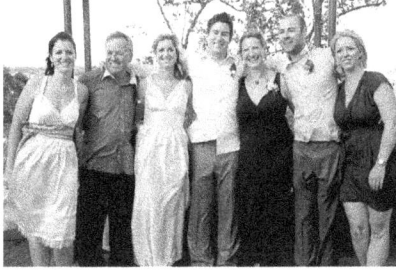

*Janey, Dad, me, Jas, Mum, Brent and Louise
on our wedding day*

Brent: *Neighsy's set-back in 2002 hasn't stopped her from doing what she loved. It hasn't kept her down. She hasn't shied away from life being deaf. She hasn't let becoming deaf hold her back, she has embraced it. It has taken her down different paths, competing for her country in deaf basketball and countless other achievements! She is one of the strongest people I know and I am proud to call her my sister. Over the years I have watched Neigh grow into a mature, thoughtful, outgoing, determined, and beautiful young lady and will always love her.*

Janey: *I find it hard to find words to explain my feelings and relationship with someone who has impacted my life in such a tremendous way. It is indescribable.*

The courage, the positivity, the strength. Renee held on and fought. Where others may have given in or up, she used all her mental strength and the power she had, to fight to come out the other side.

My view of Renee changed in all possible ways. Even to this day, fourteen years on, I look at her through precious goggles. I don't think (although she's my twin sister) she understands this. She's not perfect, she can certainly do wrong, but the way I look at her, who she is, what she does and everything in between is in a different light to before 2002.

When you come close to losing the person who has been by your side your entire life, your view will inevitably change. This could be for the short term, but for me it is long term.

I wish everyone could experience what it's like for me to hear (and what it's like for the many others affected by hearing loss – I know I'm not alone). But I can't. So often I am asked: *"What is it like? What does it sound like?"* It's a tough question to answer.

To an extent, there is no sound. I can see things but I can't hear them. It sounds like nothing except for the constant, ongoing 'buzzing' I can 'hear' known as Tinnitus. This is like a constant ringing in your ears, not the same sound as a bell, more a humming type of sound. Lots of people experience tinnitus and certainly not only deaf people. It is really hard to explain. Mum often tells me she has Tinnitus and I wonder, is it the same for her as it is for me? Do we both 'hear' the same sound? When I said it sounds like nothing, I guess that isn't exactly true – for people that can hear, using it as a comparison to describe my deafness sometimes helps.

Every other sense is enhanced to replace the missing link but it's different. You see things but you can't necessarily hear them.

I spend a large part of my life switched off, in complete silence, profoundly deaf in both ears – sometimes by choice, sometimes not. My thoughts can take over from what I might otherwise be focused on.

A common situation is for the deaf chick to say, "What was that noise?" or "What did you say?" when there's been no sound. You start hearing things that don't really exist. Ironic really.

And there are times when there is certainly a noise and I have to ask "What's that noise?" Rain on the roof, wind, an appliance; it could be anything but it's difficult for me to distinguish what the actual sound is and from where it might be coming. I hear the sound; I just have no idea what it is. This can happen thirty minutes after I've put a load of washing on, which always has the louder moments in a cycle. It's not like I have short-term memory loss or forget that I'm doing household chores, it's just that sounds appear and I don't recognise them for what they are. I'm not afraid to ask what a sound is or to ask someone to repeat themselves. And while this might cause laughter, it's not at my expense. It's because for others it's worth chuckling at someone who constantly says "sorry" or "what did you say?"

Jasey: *Renee's deafness was one of the things I loved about her when we first met, and attracted me to her. Not only was she different to most other people, but she had taken what made her different and made it an attribute rather than a disability or a hindrance. I loved that Renee was part of this whole sub-culture I knew nothing about. I was instantly motivated to learn to sign. I loved making new friends, communicating in a language I had previously known very little about, and connecting with her inspiring lifestyle.*

Living with deaf Neighsy now, after all the novelty has well and truly worn off, can be challenging at times, but I wouldn't change anything. Deafness and sign language are part of our everyday lives, and I love that. I hate that it's hard for Neighsy at times, but I love that she doesn't let it get her down. There are lots of "what?"s and "again"s (in Auslan) especially in group situations, but we make do and get by with a mixture of voice, lip-reading and signing.

Imagine being at a concert, or in a restaurant or pub where there's a huge amount of background noise and think about how difficult it is to communicate with people. You already know how hard this can be. Now try and lip-read what people are saying, keeping up with conversations. Don't be tempted to get close to their mouth or ears to yell/talk/listen – that won't help. They can't hear you and you can't hear them. Everything is muffled; nothing is clear. People talking, music, laughter – it all blends together. It's much harder to separate what you can hear than mastering and using the skill of lip-reading.

This is a common scenario and one I'm more likely to understand, as I can lip-read. It depends who is talking – different voices are more challenging than others and it can be hard work to hear what is being communicated. Over the last few months I have realised how hard I have to work to hold a conversation in these situations. Concentration on the lips that are moving over a period of time is tiring and can cause headaches. After leaving these situations, more often than not, I find the Tinnitus is really apparent and it often feels like it is contributing towards the headaches.

Picture another common scenario in my life – a hot day, riverside, sun out, sun-creamed bodies around, laughter, more freckles, cider, beer, friends, family, boats. "You're up, Neighsy!" (my turn to get into the water and behind the boat). I have to take one additional step – removing my cochlear implant to its safe haven before gearing up. *Splash!* It's gone, so for the time being, my head is underwater, my hair is wet, and I hear nothing. I'm behind the boat on my wakeboard, holding onto the handle as I glide along on top of the water (doing back flips – ha, ha, yeah, right...). Then back on the bank of the river sipping cider, reading in my lounge chair, signing every now and then, laughing.

It really doesn't seem that bad. Except that I miss most of the conversation going on, although I can see it happening, there's lots of laughter I can't relate to. I become very observant of what is happening, trying to follow conversations, occasionally asking someone who can sign what's being said. I miss heaps but it is what it is. I am there, with my friends and family having a great time. At least I am a part of the experience and am enjoying what my lifestyle has to offer.

I've lost count of the number of times people have said to me, "You're so lucky you can't hear" or "At least you don't have to listen to the boys talking rubbish". Sometimes I think, *that's easy for you to say*, but for the majority of the time that's just life for me. I can't make it different.

So yeah, my life changed a lot but I'm still known as 'derro-merro', I'm still Renee Meredith d'Offay. And while it's tough sometimes, I've learnt to live with the way it is for me. And most people around me have learnt to understand, making changes to support me. I'm more lucky than I am disadvantaged, and I keep that in my thoughts. I don't know river life any differently because I was deaf when I was introduced to the fun and started going there with Jasey.

Many people tell me I have the best of both worlds – switching off is an ability not many people have. While I had no control over what happened, deafness is never a negative thing. Challenging – yes. Difficult at times. But it's something I continue to learn to live with and embrace to ensure my life is lived to the fullest. If you dwell on the past, you forget to enjoy the future.

There are two words, however, that can be really frustrating – *don't worry*. They are the most excluding words I could hear. I naturally miss things and sometimes need to ask people to repeat themselves. I know I do this a lot, but I'm not ashamed to gain access to life around me and ensure I'm included. Some days I consciously think about how often I say "sorry" or "what" to the same person or group of people, but I won't pretend I heard if I didn't. Yes, I do need you to repeat or explain if I don't hear you, and yes, this can happen often depending on the environment. Inclusion is very important though, and is something we all need to be aware of.

There have been times where I've lacked a sense of belonging, been unsure where I fit in, stepping on eggshells so I don't make any mistakes. For an extended period of time after August 2002, I was scattered, lost, unsure what I wanted. I felt like I didn't belong. I wasn't sure where I fitted. I wasn't a part of the hearing world like I had previously been, and I'd had no exposure to the Deaf community. This was difficult to understand, but only for a short time. I built my resilience as best I could as soon as I knew how.

I felt the pressures when learning about particular opinions and beliefs some people in the Deaf community hold towards cochlear implants. At times, I took this personally because I didn't understand or know any different. As time went by, I began to understand where this defensive and strong opinion comes from.

My understanding now is that the majority of the Deaf community don't 'hate' people who have cochlear implants, they're just genuinely concerned about what will happen to the unique and important aspects of their community and culture such as Auslan (Australian Sign Language) if many deaf people are implanted and choose to communicate with spoken language. Of course, this can be personal for some people but it highlights the importance of professionals, including hospitals and clinics, promoting ALL the avenues available and providing patients with a range of information.

My family and I were not given any information about the Deaf community or sign language when my life changed – information that I now feel is very important, especially for young children and their families.

Families should be provided with the information, support and understanding they need to help make their own decisions. I've found that it's common to label children and adults as 'signing deaf' or 'oral deaf', which I think contributes towards the mixed theories people like myself might feel, and social connectedness for young adults. Being able to adjust to change or accept situations the way they are can be difficult, and outside pressure can be hard of individuals and families. From my personal experience and work in educational environments, one of the most important areas of exposure and understanding for young children and adults is giving each of them the ability to create their own sense of identity, regardless of their abilities.

Sometimes we do or say things we don't realise might have an impact on others. We are all guilty of this. Working to dissolve the boundaries and separation between minority groups and becoming an accepting, comfortable and collaborative place to live is something we all want. For ourselves. For each other. But most importantly, for our future generations.

I was introduced to Danny, the first deaf person I had ever met, during my recovery period in 2002 by mutual friends. Danny was born deaf to deaf parents and had grown up communicating in Auslan. Growing up in Geelong, I can't recall seeing deaf people out in the community. My only knowledge of deafness was of old people getting hearing aids because they were, well... old.

As I was still learning to lip-read and had no idea about Auslan, we communicated by writing to each other on a note pad. I still remember this day so well. I was very nervous, butterflies in my tummy – all for no reason, of course. This was an opportunity for Danny to share his experiences with me, helping me to understand what his life has been like growing up in a deaf family as well as my chance to ask questions and learn about some of his experiences to help ease my misunderstandings and curiosity.

Every day there were so many new questions. I was anxious about saying the wrong things, though I was soon able to start joining some of the dots of the life I had entered. Danny eased some of my initial concerns and answered my questions in a very casual and friendly way. Although his story was very different to mine, it was reassuring to feel some kind of connection after such a massive change. I'm thankful to my friends for introducing me to Danny that day. It opened a door for me to meet many more wonderful people just like him.

For a long time, every time I met a deaf person, I felt as if I had to impress them, give reasoning behind the decisions I had made and what I had been through. When I began learning Auslan, I was nervous signing to fluent Auslan users and often made mistakes, which made me more nervous and less confident. There came a time when I realised I was the only one judging me and I just needed to relax, be myself, regardless of who I was talking to.

Once I accepted this, I started to discover and feel my sense of belonging. I felt as if I could sit in the middle of a Venn diagram; I'm part of both worlds – hearing and deaf, in the section where they overlap. I started creating my own space where I didn't necessarily have to belong here or there. With practice and persistence, I've stopped trying to fit into one or the other and just let it be.

And now people come into my shared space and we have so much fun. We sign-dance nights away to old school tunes, we prepare each other for good and bad times, and we just live each day as if it's the last as often as we can.

I've had my hands in so many baskets, been greedy some might say. I have degrees, qualifications, certificates and diplomas in a wide range of fields, and each has become a part of a created piece of the puzzle I call 'Neighsy's Life'.

The loss of my natural hearing presented some side effects that contribute to some funny memories. For example, my balance was affected. For the first two weeks of recovery, I needed the support of walls or someone's strength to walk with because without them I either fell down or looked drunk! That's a pretty big deal for anyone, but for a nineteen-year-old, independent woman it was more than annoying having to rely on others for support. I couldn't drive, couldn't walk.

I clearly remember celebrating to myself, then proudly sharing it with EVERYONE, the day I walked alone and started regaining my independence. These small milestones were all a part of my journey to recovery. My balance now is still far from the way it was prior to 2002, like my ability to hear. But I manage. I'm used to things the way they are.

When it's dark I find it harder to keep my balance, as I can't see as well to focus on the surface I'm on. I often step out of line or walk into people. And it doesn't have to be dark for me to occasionally override my step. Most people are used to this and say nothing. Other times I have to apologise for my incorrect walking. So be it. It's not a big deal.

I've been Deaf now for over fourteen years, and I will be forever. Accepting that and living with it daily has been challenging, rewarding and everything you can find in-between.

CHAPTER EIGHT

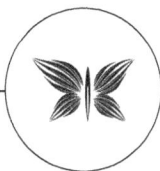

Dealing with loss and grief

Most of us at some point in our lives have experienced loss followed shortly by grief. Most of us have become familiar with what it's like to go through challenges that are out of our control, that have an impact on the way we look at life, the decisions we make, how we feel. Sometimes other people's experiences have an impact on us and how we feel. At other times, the impact is direct – straight to oneself.

There have been rare occasions when I've felt sad while I wonder what people are saying, what sounds things are making. When I've thought about what I'm missing out on. Sometimes I've wished for my life to be different – like it was before, but rarely.

But it isn't a matter of pushing away these feelings for me. It's more they haven't entered my mind very often. Is this because of my approach and acceptance and understanding of what happened? Is it due to my personality and positive attitude? Or, have I learnt how to grieve? Then come the questions – *Was I already like this? Or, is this the person I have become? What would my life have been like if it hadn't been turned upside down all those years ago?*

Over time, with hours of professional help, I have learnt that grief is as important as other emotions, reactions, and the recovery process. Sweeping your feelings under the rug is not the best approach, but this is something we don't always realise we're doing. I got on with life without really considering how big a loss I had experienced. I went back to work as soon as I could and carried on in the way I always had.

After ten years, it became clear – although it had to be pointed out to me – that I had failed to mourn my loss. My natural hearing was gone forever and I was too busy being positive and supported, I forgot to grieve. Maybe I hadn't pushed anything away, but I also hadn't let it in. Things were a lot different, permanently. I felt, knew, and accepted this, but I hadn't taken the time to recognise the sad aspects of what had happened.

In some ways this loss was like any other loss that occurs in people's lives, but in other ways it was very different. I went from nineteen years of hearing to complete deafness – a huge loss! I hope this is the biggest loss I'll have to experience, although I know there will be more to come during my life.

As humans, we are unique individuals with our own emotions, personalities and choices. Losing one of the five senses most people live with their whole life has certainly changed the person I was, but it's also helped shape who I am and who I want to be.

As well as loss, it has also given me so much – friendships, strength, a different outlook, motivation, determination and much, much more. Not being able to change the way I am now has a big influence on me not trying to. I can't, so I won't, but if I could, would I? I believe I have found other things to try to control and many more things I can't.

I don't hold this event entirely responsible for helping me understand grief. I'm thirty-four years old, so I'm naturally learning and growing with age and through experience. All my life experiences have contributed towards the person I am, my beliefs and my actions. I'm grateful I have discovered aspects of mental health I didn't understand, and that have helped me to deal with loss differently and allow grief to come and go as expected. *If it comes, let it; if it goes, let it.*

Loss is not a competition. For me, it's been about the journey of dealing with loss and grief rather than focusing on them, weaving them into my life.

During a recent difficult time, a very wise man gave me a different perspective and attitude towards life. His description involved thinking of life as a piece of cloth where different threads are woven together. When a thread comes loose, rather than focusing on it and potentially pulling it out, thread it back through the material. In life, that loose thread represents a difficult situation, one where grief would be expected. Rather than focusing on grieving until it passes because this may never happen, weave the grief through the rest of your life. In time, you might grieve again over the same experience. However, it is part of the cloth, part of your life.

Sadly, at the end of 2015, Jason and I lost our first baby. It came as a complete shock at our twelve week scan and left us both literally speechless in a room together for half an hour. I used my strength and positivity to reflect on the situation that was out of our control, but this time things were different. I also allowed myself to grieve.

I got through some really hard times with deep, uncontrollable crying, often not knowing exactly why. And Jason just held me in his arms, saying nothing or telling me it was OK. Him holding me was enough. We connected like never before, and this took our relationship and friendship to a different level.

My beautiful family and friends were there for me again. I drove straight from the room of silence to Mum and Dad's and walked directly into Mum's arms where she held me as I sobbed telling her. I dealt with this heart-breaking situation as best I could by allowing myself to grieve. There were nine days straight of me seriously grieving the loss and feeling the sorrow. During this time I completed my first year at the big school, had my birthday (without Janey), and Christmas.

Of course, there was plenty of happiness and laughter, but underlying all of that, the sense of loss was so raw, so close. After sharing our news with close family and friends, we realised just how common miscarriages can be, and this helped us to understand and slowly move forward. It's true that time can contribute towards healing.

In May, 2016, Jas and I learnt we were pregnant again. However, this time we approached the situation differently. We didn't say much to many people, waiting cautiously as we approached the twelve week scan, hoping for a better outcome than before. At the twelve week scan we were lucky enough to see what we hadn't six months earlier, a heartbeat. Unfortunately, there was fluid (foetal hydrops) under the baby's skin and in its chest cavity, so again it wasn't a positive ultrasound. With not much more to go on, we were told it was most likely an infection that would pass and to wait until sixteen weeks for another scan. It was the longest month of our lives.

The next weeks involved lots more waiting and a range of tests to eliminate possible causes of the hydrops. We were told every time we went to an appointment that they were surprised the baby had made it as far as it had – and we were heartbroken. At twenty-three weeks gestation, I went into an induced labour to give birth to our deceased baby boy, who never got to experience a day of life.

Now I am even more thankful for understanding grief, and I can be gentle and kind to myself as I try to understand such a horrible situation. The grief remains; there are constant reminders of my loss all around me. But as I learnt to weave the threads by making the most of what I have learnt, of what I know, the grief slowly changes. There is no formula to deal with loss. We are all very different individuals, and when loss creates change, you can make some choices around that material you have woven.

The good and bad things we experience often have an impact on the people around us, not just ourselves. Being kind and thoughtful to others is important as everyone deals with grief and loss differently, and the better we understand this, the more successful our support can be. We never know what people might be going through or may have experienced. And I truly can't emphasise enough how much I believe that everything happens for a reason.

CHAPTER NINE

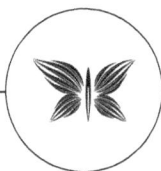

Here and beyond

Like with all important dates and anniversaries, each year as the middle of August approaches my emotions start changing. For the first couple of years, and also on the ten year anniversary, we made a strong effort to recognise and celebrate the positive outcome of a life-changing event. We celebrated less in other years, but have always appreciated that this date is a significant time to reflect on life and on changing.

I love my life the way it is. We had dinner with friends this year, a high school friend and her husband who are a great support to Jason and me – we find them inspirational. As we were talking it occurred to me that there were so many things about my story this friend didn't know. While I'd shared some information, mostly about my ability to hear things and my life with my cochlear, I told them I didn't want to let the cat out of the bag. They had waited this long to hear my story, I figured a little longer and they could share my experience through reading my book.

There are many people who know me well – family and friends – but some of them don't *really* know me. Not only am I sharing my story with friends, family and complete strangers, my book has given me the opportunity to share it with the world! I am so excited and very motivated by this. Writing and sharing my book is part of a dream come true.

With motivation, confidence and support, if you set out to achieve your goals and dreams, it's likely that at some stage success will follow. I'm in the very early stages of this, and things might not work out like I've planned, but I'm determined and guided by the inspiration of others to give it a really good go. Of course, there will be more challenges – you're crazy if you think your life will never be complicated. But I've tackled different and unexpected challenges over the last fifteen years, and I want to help others feel like they are not alone. I want to continue to soar, continue to learn and inspire. I'm a blessed individual and hugely grateful for such a supported, positive life.

If my book is read by a hundred people and inspires one, my goal will be achieved. If I stand in a classroom, on a stage or in front of an audience to share my story and one person is inspired, I will have been successful. We all have a story worth sharing. I hope that by reading mine, you can feel and see that life can change when you least expect it.

Accept and support change. Get on with what life presents, and how it allows you to be the best possible version of yourself. Be proud of yourself and create happiness within. Above all, be open to change and willing to make a difference in your own life.

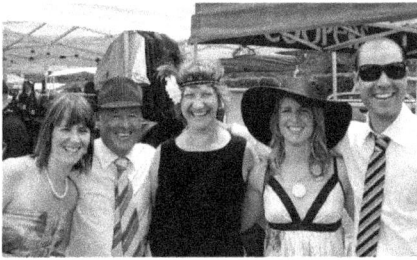

*Janey, Roysie, Bettsy, me and Brent enjoying
a family day at the races. I love you all unconditionally
no matter what – thank you .*

Justin's
DOUBLE
DELIGHT
In SPORT

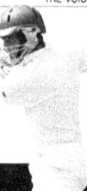

Super
crossword
Book and
movie reviews

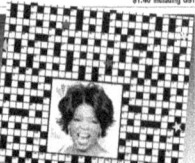

In today's BIG WEEKEND magazine

MENINGOCOCCAL NIGHTMARE

LEARNING TO HEAR AGAIN

NATALIE STAAKS

RENEE Kahle was plunged into an eerie world of silence when meningococcal disease robbed her of her hearing overnight.

But the Breamlea 20-year-old knows she is lucky to be alive after surviving the deadly bug four months ago.

"I look at myself and I think I could've died," she said yesterday.

"I'd rather have lost my hearing than an arm or a leg."

On August 9 this year Renee woke up feeling nauseous and was diagnosed with a simple virus.

The next day she was deaf.

"I woke up and my head was killing and I yelled out and I couldn't hear myself," she said.

It is unknown how she contracted the disease or what strain of the bug it was.

"As far as I'm concerned I was living my normal life and I'm never going to know how it happened — that's one of the annoying things, I'll never know," Renee said.

She spent two days in intensive care and a week in Geelong Hospital with her identical twin sister Jane never leaving her side.

Three months to the day Renee contracted the killer bug she was given a bionic ear.

She was "switched on" to the world on October 28, able to hear again after months of lip reading and writing messages on a whiteboard.

"It's nothing like natural hearing, it's really hard to explain," Renee said.

"I've had to teach myself to hear again. It will always be like that, that's just the hearing I have."

Renee said the decision to get a bionic ear implant was a difficult one as the operation wipes out all natural hearing.

But doctors believed the bones in her ears were so damaged she would never regain her natural hearing.

"I'm really lucky that I had the chance to hear for 19 years," she said.

"In so many ways I'm so lucky and in other ways I wish it had been put off for another five years."

Renee is a third-year apprentice hairdresser whose love of life was heightened by her brush with meningococcal.

Her aim is to travel and go snowboarding in Canada although she is unsure if that will be possible as her illness not only affected her hearing.

"I lost all my balance too, I looked drunk," she said.

CONTINUED Page 2

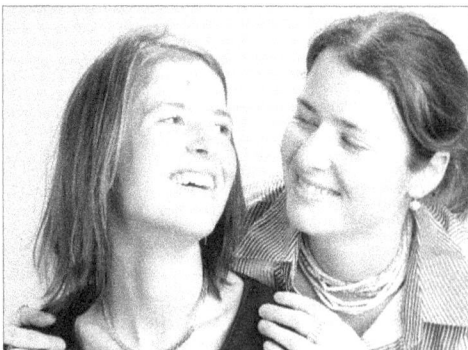

SWITCHED ON: Renee Kahle, left, can hear her twin sister Jane again thanks to the bionic ear Renee had implanted after her fight with the shocking meningococcal disease.
Photo: MIKE DUGDALE

WEATHER   Fine apart from early morning fog. Top: 27. Details page 39.   CONTACTS   General: 5227 4300 Classifieds: 131 585 Internet: www.geelonginfo.com

Learning to Hear Again - Saturday 28th December, 2002.
Front Cover. Courtesy of The Geelong Advertiser.

welcome to

Geelong Advertiser

| SATURDAY, DECEMBER 28, 2002

Monday

in the know

In The Know is your daily lifestyle guide covering food, gardening, fashion, health, technology and fun.
Don't miss it. Monday to Friday in your Geelong Advertiser!

Coming up

MONDAY	TUESDAY	WEDNESDAY	THURSDAY
SPORTING ROUNDUP			weddings

tattslotto

POWERBALL: Draw No. 345
26, 9, 5, 10, 8. Powerball: 2.
Dividends: Div 1 jackpots.
Div 2 $46,202.65; Div 3 $4493.90;
Div 4 $76.95; Div 5 $32.55;
Div 6 $19.10; Div 7 $8.05.
TATTS TWO: 90, 81.
Dividend $8.31.
KENO: 1, 2, 6, 13, 17, 18, 21, 23, 24, 25, 26, 28, 49, 62, 64, 66, 70, 74, 77, 79.
No Spot 10 winner. Jackpots to $1,073,800.

WHERE TO FIND US

GENERAL
phone: **5227 4300** fax: 5227 4330

CLASSIFIEDS
phone (local call): **131 586**
email: classifieds@geelongadvertiser.com.au

NEWS
phone: 5227 4351 fax: 5227 4342
email: pcmo@geelongadvertiser.com.au

SPORT
phone: 5227 4368 fax: 5227 4342
email: sport@geelongadvertiser.com.au

ADVERTISING
phone: 5227 4350 fax: 5227 4385
email: advert@geelongadvertiser.com.au

NEWSPAPER DELIVERY
phone (free call): 1800 353 734
email: circulation@geelongadvertiser.com.au

GEELONG NEWS and THE ECHO
phone: 5227 4417 fax: 5227 4428
email: newscollar@geelongadvertiser.com.au

Printed and published at 61 Leaflet Street, Breakwater, 3219 for the Geelong Advertiser Proprietary Limited, 191-195 Ryrie Street, Geelong 3220. Telephone (03) 5227 4300. Fax (03) 5227 4330. ABN 59 004 080 055.

Sewerage plant birds' haven

FOR people, the rank-smelling sewage treatment plant at Werribee is the city's largest drain, infamous for its hydrogen sulphide pong.

For birds, it's a bit like paradise.

Every summer thousands of migratory waders from Siberia, Alaska and Asia fly up to 12,000 kilometres to escape the harsh northern winter and revel in the smelly wetlands.

Victoria Wader Study Group volunteers yesterday netted and banded 200 of the red-necked stint species, which had recently arrived from breeding grounds in northeastern Siberia.

The group will today focus on netting two other wader species that make the six to eight week journey, the sharp-tailed sandpiper and the curlew sandpiper.

The birds fly for two to three days at a time for stretches of up to 5000 kilometres.

Group leader Dr Clive Minton said the 10,851 hectare site, on the shores of Port Phillip Bay, was an ideal summer vacation spot for waders because it provided a rich source of food.

"There are mudflats and sand flats which at low tide are very rich in worms and

shellfish," Dr Minton said.

"As the tide comes in they can go onto Melbourne Water's sewage ponds which provide more food and shelter."

The Victorian Wader Study Group nets and bands the birds every year as part of a worldwide effort to monitor their migratory movements, survival and reproduction rates.

sewerspill

Smelly end to holiday

PETER BEGG

IT didn't take a Grovedale family of six long to realise what was bubbling from a vent just outside their back door about 9pm on Boxing Day.

Raw sewage!

And within minutes both indoor toilets and the shower drain hole were also spewing forth raw sewage throughout the house.

By the time the State Emergency Service arrived, within six minutes of being called, the Grovedale house had about 15

centimetres of raw sewerage covering the floors.

Staff from Barwon Water arrived shortly afterwards, and advised the problem was with a blocked sewer main nearby.

The Grovedale family's house just happened to be the first house 'upstream' from the blockage. No other houses were affected.

Two SES units and 10 volunteers turned up at the Grovedale address, where they activated the sewerage release valves to the house. They also placed sandbags in front of areas of the house not already affected

by the flood and helped remove household valuables.

The family was evacuated to a relative's house, and the City of Greater Geelong was yesterday arranging emergency accommodation.

The Grovedale couple returned to the house yesterday, where the damage was being calculated by an insurance assessor.

The couple, who preferred not to be identified, said the smell did not have to be described.

The father described how he virtually had a Pine

O Cleen shower afterwards.

The mother was philosophical, and said at least it didn't happen on Christmas Day in the middle of their festive lunch.

Meanwhile, several houses in Geelong West were without water on Christmas night after a water service pipe burst in Candover Street.

One Geelong West couple arrived home about midnight to find Barwon Water workers on site.

A spokesman said the water was back on within the hour.

Price rise

The price of Saturday's Geelong Advertiser will increase by 10 cents next week.

The new price of the Saturday Advertiser will be $1.50, including GST.

The Monday to Friday price will remain unchanged.

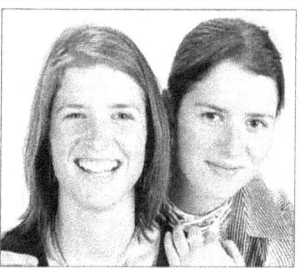

TIME TO SMILE: Renee and Kane Kahle have good reason to be happy after Renee survived her fight with meningococcal disease.

Renee learns to hear again

FROM Page 1

"I was so proud one day when I didn't need anyone's help (to walk) and it just picked up from there."

Meningococcal is commonly spread through saliva.

Renee said she was now a "drinks Nazi" if she saw her friends sharing drinks.

She has also urged her friends to get vaccinated against the disease, as she, twin Jane and older brother Brent have been.

"I can't make people do it, I wish I could," she said.

"Everyone was so shocked, you never expect it to happen to you or someone so close.

"You just don't realise how special you are."

*Learning to Hear Again - Saturday 28th December, 2002. Pg 2.
Courtesy of The Geelong Advertiser.*

Man killed dog with axe

Renee shoots for China

MICHAELA FARRINGTON

DEADLY meningococcal disease robbed Renee Kahle of her hearing four years ago, plunging her into a world of silence.

But neither the deadly illness nor losing her hearing could dent Ms Kahle's determination to live an extraordinary life.

Now the 23-year-old is preparing for her next challenge — competing at the World Deaf Basketball Championships in China next year.

Ms Kahle was recently selected for the Australian Women's Deaf Basketball team and will travel with her teammates to the world championships in June, if they can raise the funds or find sponsors to help get them there.

Four years ago, Ms Kahle's life was very different.

She was a 19-year-old apprentice hairdresser when meningococcal meningitis struck.

Ms Kahle woke one morning with a splitting headache and a churning stomach.

She dragged herself out of bed and went to work, not realising she had contracted a life-threatening disease.

She was rushed to hospital the next day, in agony and unable to hear.

But Ms Kahle doesn't spend much time looking back on that time of pain and fear when she spent three nights in intensive care, and woke to a different life.

"It was pretty scary," Ms Kahle said. "It took a while to hit home.

"I still have bad days,

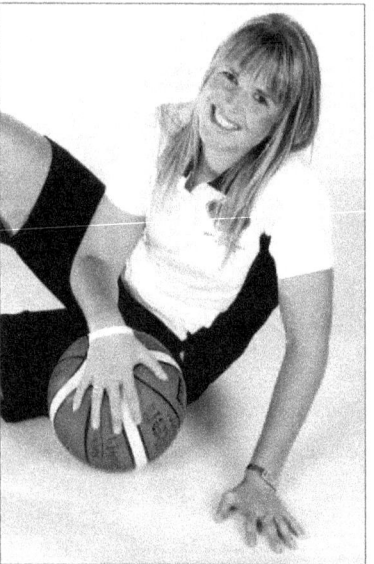

but "And so much has come out of it."

Three months after she contracted meningococcal, Ms Kahle was given a bionic ear implant and learned to hear again.

"I'm looking forward, not back," Ms Kahle

said, "And so much has come out of it."

One of the things Ms Kahle is looking forward to is competing in front of her home-town crowd when Geelong hosts the National Deaf Basketball Club Championships in April.

In the meantime, she is busy drumming up support for her team, training with her national and state teammates and working three jobs.

One of Ms Kahle many jobs is working as a communication aid

for 13 deaf children at Grovedale West Primary School.

She has spent two years studying sign language full time while losing her hearing and has applied to study teaching next year. She hopes to one day teach deaf children.

HOOPS HOPE: Renee Kahle, who lost her hearing after contracting meningococcal four years ago, has earned a place on the national women's deaf basketball team and will be competing in China next year. Photo: GLENN FERGUSON

KAREN MATTHEWS

WITNESSES watched in horror as a man bludgeoned a dog to death with an axe after it was hit by a car, a court has heard.

Pleas by the witnesses to be allowed to get assistance for the injured animal were ignored as the dog's owner Adam Martinko allowed his neighbour Geoffrey Farington to repeatedly hit the injured animal.

Farington, 62, and Martinko, 38, both of Neil St, Bell Post Hill, appeared in Geelong Magistrates' Court yesterday. Farington pleaded guilty to beating an animal and Martinko pleaded guilty to failing to provide treatment for an injured animal.

RSPCA prosecutor Jason Nichols said the charges arose from an incident in July when Martinko's dog was hit by a car in Neil St, Bell Post Hill.

He said despite being just five minutes from North Geelong Veterinary Clinic, Martinko allowed Farington to kill the dog.

Mr Nichol said distressed witnesses pleaded to be allowed to get assistance.

He said witnesses also told RSPCA inspectors that the dog yelped when the first blow landed, contradicting claims by

Farington and Martinko that the dog was unconscious at the time.

The prosecutor said inspectors investigated after receiving distressing calls about the incident.

"When they arrived inspectors followed a trail of blood to a back yard where they exhumed the dog's body," he said.

"A post mortem revealed the dog had been repeatedly beaten to the front of the head with a small axe and this would have caused suffering to the animal."

Mary Foley, for Farington and Martinko, said her clients' regarded the act as necessary in the circumstances.

She said Farington saw her neighbour in distress and acted to help his friend.

"Mr Farington comes from a farm background where you don't wait for the vet," Ms Foley said.

"Mr Martinko was grief-stricken when the dog was hit by a car and it was because of his grief that he acted that way."

Magistrate Ian von Einem said the dog should have been taken to the vet and treated properly, stressing it was not the way its animals to be put down.

Farington and Martinko were convicted and each fined $750 with $125 costs.

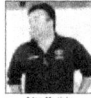

Adam Martinko

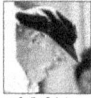

Geoffrey Farington

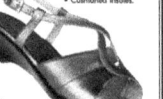

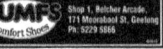

New mayor decided tonight

REBECCA TUCKER

THE State Government has ruled out granting Geelong a direct election of the city's mayor.

And it will not extend terms beyond one year as Geelong councillors tonight vote in their fifth leader since March, 2002.

During the same time, and longer, City of Melbourne Lord Mayor John So has been in power, popularly elected in July 2001.

Cr So was yesterday voted the world's most popular mayor.

And in Ballarat, Mayor David Vendy will tonight be elected for a seventh consecutive term, after also beginning his term in 2001.

All of Geelong's four most recent mayors, Barbara Abley, Ed Coppe, Shane Dowling and incumbent Peter McMullin, have in the past called for the people to elect the city's leader for four-year terms.

The agitation from within the council ranks has been supported by lobby group the Committee for Geelong.

And the Liberal Party

made a popular mayor for Geelong a policy during the election campaign.

But the Government has refused the calls.

"We have no plans to change the current system," a spokeswoman for incoming Local Government Minister Richard Wynne said.

Geelong's next mayor is widely tipped to be Cr Bruce Harwood, in a deal believed to have been set up some time ago.

Ballarat Mayor David Vendy, Victoria's longest serving mayor, said the community was the

biggest winner of longer terms.

He said it took at least one year to learn the job and set things in place for the long term.

But changing the leader on a yearly basis created inconsistency and instability.

"The job sounds easy but it's not that simple," Cr Vendy said.

Ballarat also has one year terms but Cr Vendy said he consistently won the support of the majority of the nine-member council by keeping personal and party politics out of the job.

X-rated X-ray sparks outcry

A NEW full-body X-ray machine which shows graphic images of nude bodies will be tested at a US airport this month.

The Backscatter machine has brought an outcry from civil rights advocates who claim the technology amounts to a virtual strip search.

"This doesn't only concern genitals but body size, body shape and other things like evidence of mastectomies, colostomy appliances or catheter tubes," privacy expert Jay Stanley said.

Woman jailed for conning priest, 83

Panel to decide planning zones

PETER BEGG

DANIEL FOGARTY

A GAMBLING-ADDICTED "predator" who conned an elderly Melbourne Catholic priest into handing over his life savings has been jailed.

Olivia Raymond used fake documents and said stories to trick 83-year-old Fr Paul Kane into handing over $400,000 from accounts belonging to St Matthew's Parish in the northern Melbourne suburb of Fawkner.

She also conned the priest out of nearly $50,000 of his own money - savings for his retirement.

Raymond gambled away all the money on poker machines.

Victorian County Court Judge Howard Mason yesterday said Raymond's actions would not only make the priest's retirement harder, but also affect members of the community who relied on the church for charity.

"You exhausted the life savings of a vulnerable and compassionate elderly man," Judge Mason said.

"These are serious crimes. Your actions were calculated, cruel and predatory."

Raymond, 31, of Epping, pleaded guilty to five counts of obtaining property by deception and one count of making a false document.

Judge Mason jailed her for four years and eight months.

The court heard Raymond used excuses including stories about the death of her mother, who was in court yesterday, and cancer surgery.

She told the "unworldly" priest that she had won the lottery and would soon receive more than $200,000.

The court heard the deception began in 2005 when Raymond approached the priest upset and asking for cash.

The priest gave her $20.

Raymond returned and began asking regularly for cash.

The sophistication of her designs increased and she began using fake letters, false loans documents and forged cheques.

In one note she wrote: "Three guys have tortured my

life. They broke into my house and trashed it."

In another she said: "Father Paul, I understand what you have said about no cash in accounts I have broken promise after promise to you. I am aware of the figure please trust me."

She urged him to give her $8,500 and put an end to it, saying "I will never knock on your door again."

Raymond must serve two and a half years in prison before being eligible for parole.

— AAP

THE area of central Geelong to be subject to a controversial Development Assessment Committee will be decided by an independent panel.

This is one of several changes to the Development Assessment Committee forced on the State Government after its original legislation was defeated in the Upper House in June.

New legislation is expected to go before parliament this week.

Development Assessment Committees will make planning permit decisions over designated areas in conjunction with local government.

The Victorian Liberal Nationals Coalition added the new legislation included valuable safeguards for local communities.

Liberal planning spokesman Matthew Guy said the changes included:

LIMITING committees to only 26 principal activity centres, including Geelong;

FORCING the Brumby Government to consult with relevant local government associations when choosing the chairperson for each committee;

REMOVING the requirement of councils to cover the direct costs of the committees;

FORCING committee operational areas to be decided by an independent panel recommendation to the minister; and

REQUIRING an independent planning panel to set the recommended trigger points for each committee after consultation with the community and the relevant municipality.

Geelong councillor Andrew Katos said he spoke to a Sydney delegate at the recent Cities in Transition conference in Geelong who had experienced difficulties with a similar program being implemented in New South Wales.

Geelong to host Australian Deaf Games in 2012

GEELONG is fast gaining a name for itself as host of elite sporting competitions, securing yet another national sporting event.

The city will host the 16th Australian Deaf Games in early 2012, after making a successful bid for the multi-sport event, which is likely to attract 1000 participants and up to 1500 support staff

Geelong out-bid Wodonga to secure the event following a tour by organisers of the city's sports and other facilities.

"It's all about being able to hold the event successfully and Geelong has proved it can do that with the other events it has hosted," City of Greater Geelong councillor Bruce Harwood said.

"Our wide range of high quality sports facilities including the Arena, Kardinia Pool, Landy Field and Geelong Baseball Centre played a big part in securing this national event. And we're not a capital city so it means it doesn't cost as much for event organisers.

"And we have huge acceptance from the community which is always key to a successful event."

Held every four years, the Games involve up to 20 different sports and attract competitors from all over Australia and New Zealand.

Geelong's Renee Kahle, a member of the Australian Women's Deaf Basketball team, said she was thrilled the event was coming to her home town.

"This is my first time to participate in this event and I'm so excited it's so close to home," she said.

"Geelong is an awesome place to host Australian Deaf Games, with great facilities and a supportive community. I'm sure lots of people will be keen to get involved."

The Australian Deaf Games is one of the oldest sporting events in the country.

The origins of interstate deaf sport competitions can be traced back to 1896 when the Victorian Deaf Cricket team travelled to South Australia for a friendly cricket match.

The first Deaf Carnivale were held in 1611 and continued regularly until the Games in its current format started in 1964. The most recent Games were held on the Gold Coast in January 2009.

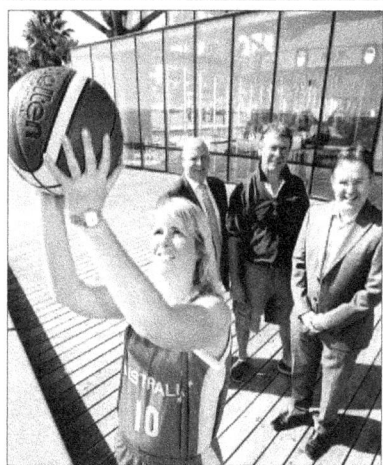

GAMES ON: Joining basketballer Renee Kahle yesterday to announce Geelong's successful bid to host the games was Mayor John Mitchell, events portfolio holder Bruce Harwood and Chairman of Australian Deaf Games Richard Pearce.

City wins on safety

THE City of Greater Geelong has won an award for a program designed to increase children's safety in the region.

The City won the Local Government Category of the Australian Safer Communities Awards for its SafeStart Project, which aims to work with communities to stop preventable injuries from occurring.

Community development portfolio holder councillor Kylie Fisher said the program had helped make Geelong a safer place to live.

"The development of the SafeStart Project has helped to create a healthier and safer environment for local children and thereby for the whole community," Cr Fisher said.

Time to have say on Drysdale's future

TONY PRYTZ

A NEW round of public consultation on the Drysdale Clifton Springs structure plan will start on Monday, city councillor Rod Macdonald said this week.

The wide-ranging plan has caused some concern with locals but Cr Macdonald said now was the time for people to have their say.

The plan envisages a major overhaul of the Drysdale central area with provision for new supermarkets, improved footpaths, bike tracks and restructured sporting facilities.

The co-ordinator of the Springdale Neighbourhood Centre, Ann Brackley, said as it stood the plan replaced the centre's child care service with a car park.

"It shows half our buildings are to be pulled down and replaced by car park," she said.

Ms Brackley said she could not believe the council would do that.

"Not after we spent $1 million on the centre only a few years ago," she said

"I don't understand why they put that in the structure plan."

But Cr Rod McDonald said the document was not finalised.

"These things are concept plans and more work needs to be done before the final plan is developed," he said.

"The (Springdale) cen-

tre will not lose any services. The plan is to improve services."

Cr Macdonald encouraged anyone with concerns or views on the future of the area to have a say during the consultation period.

Drysdale Bowling and Croquet Club director Lex Mortimer said members were still waiting for more detail about the proposal for the club to be relocated.

"We still have to get a majority of club members

in favour of the move," he said.

Mr Mortimer said he initially favoured the move but as time went on people's enthusiasm had waned.

"We are no further advanced than we were 18 months ago," he said.

He said the delays meant some people, including himself, were "getting cold on the idea".

Cr Macdonald said while there had been action behind the scenes,

funding to commence planning for the move was not available until this council budget.

"That project will be starting very soon," he said.

"We have to come up with a plan for the club's future."

Cr Macdonald said co-location of sporting clubs had to be considered.

"The sporting club at Lara has eight sporting bodies using the one facility," he said.

Geelong to host the Australian Deaf Games in 2012 - Thursday 12th November, 2009, pg 16. Courtesy of The Geelong Advertiser.

Jab would be a lifesaver - Saturday 4th February, 2017, Pg 14. Courtesy of The Geelong Advertiser.

Acknowledgments

I would not be here to write this book, and my story would not have been successful or near as powerful without these beautiful humans.

Mum and Dad – Betty and Roy.

My twin sister – Jane/Janey.

My brother – Brent.

My husband and soul mate – Jason/Jasey/Jas.

Their contribution to all aspects of my life make me, ME! I am forever grateful to them for pulling me through my darkest hours and believing in me.

To **Nicole Love, Michelle d'Offay, and Louise Kahle**– my sisters-in-law–thank you for encouraging me and supporting my life.

Special mention to **Janey and Nic** for introducing me to Jasey, you led me to the only guy I want to spend the rest of my life with, big nose and all.

My writing focus group, the team of friends, colleagues and students who took the time to read sections of my book during the writing process.

Ann-Marie Mullen-Walsh

Robert Walker

Cody Pettina

Madeline Lewis

Nat, Kal, Laura and **Macka Heard**

Sally Martin, for being a huge part of my life since losing my hearing, and in particular in my career in deaf education. It was through her connections I found Julie and her encouragement to make my story a reality for everyone to share. Thank you.

Danny Ashley, the first Deaf person to whom I was introduced, and who has had a big influence on my understanding and ability to transition between the two communities.

Mary Mavrias, my 'advocate', for her support and encouragement.

Julie Postance, book publishing consultant, mentor, and positive role model.

Kate Toholka, mentor and all-round lover of successful women.

Lindsay Gardiner, my friend, my motivator, photographer, inspiration, and contributor to my success.

Jane Blakston, my dearly supportive friend.

Maureen Hoare, for contributing to our welcoming into this world that made life much less stressful for Mum and Dad. Thank you.

David Pereira, a man of knowledge who has supported my ability to weave my life.

Lauren and Tim Davies, for their belief in good things, their motivation to keep things real, and for their wisdom.

Xaiver Rudd, for telling me very early on that I had a story to be published.

To all my dear family and friends, it's because of each of you – at different times in my life – that I found the passion to share my story. I truly am a very lucky individual to have experienced a challenging life but have barely felt alone. May each of you recognise your importance in my life.

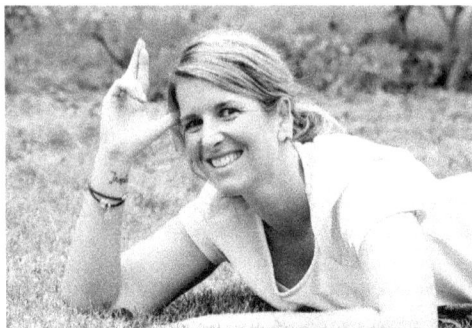

About the Author

Renee d'Offay is an inspiring Deaf role model who has touched the hearts of many through sharing her challenging experiences. She is a qualified Teacher of the Deaf, and LOTE Auslan teacher living in Geelong, Australia, with her husband Jason, and their dog, Ouzo.

Renee was born thirteen minutes before her twin sister Jane on December 22, 1982. She grew up with her family in the small Victorian coastal town of Breamlea. Renee was born and lived with natural hearing for nineteen years before she contracted meningococcal meningitis in 2002, which left her profoundly deaf. This life-changing experience encouraged Renee to have a new outlook on life, and started her on a journey for which she could never be prepared.

Renee d'Offay – who is known by family and friends as 'Neighsy' – has written this book to share her life experiences, struggles, and opportunities after losing all natural hearing in both her ears. With this book, Renee hopes her audience will find some inspiration and motivation within their own lives, as well as an understanding as to what it can be like to deal with loss and life's unexpected challenges.

www.ingramcontent.com/pod-product-compliance
Lightning Source LLC
Chambersburg PA
CBHW020301030426
42336CB00010B/852